Contents

CW01500349

Multiple Orgasms in Groups

Riding the Wave in Group Scenarios

O Maxima

ISBN: 9781778905001
Imprint: Telephasic Workshop
Copyright © 2024 O Maxima.
All Rights Reserved.

Introduction

Understanding the Potential of Group Sexual Encounters

Exploring the Taboo: Why Group Sex is a Popular Fantasy

Group sex, often shrouded in societal taboos, emerges as a powerful fantasy for many individuals. This allure can be traced to various psychological, social, and biological factors that intertwine to create an enticing narrative of pleasure, freedom, and exploration. Understanding why group sex captivates the imagination requires delving into the complexities of human sexuality and the cultural narratives that shape our desires.

The Psychology of Taboo

At its core, the appeal of group sex lies in its taboo nature. Sigmund Freud's theories on repression suggest that societal constraints often heighten desires for what is forbidden. The thrill of engaging in a sexual experience that defies conventional norms can evoke a sense of liberation and empowerment. This is particularly relevant in a culture where monogamy is often idealized, making the idea of multiple partners both exhilarating and forbidden.

The concept of *forbidden fruit* plays a significant role here. When something is deemed taboo, it often becomes more desirable. This phenomenon can be explained by the *reactance theory*, which posits that individuals experience a negative emotional response when they perceive their freedoms being restricted. Consequently, the allure of group sex can be seen as a form of rebellion against societal norms, allowing individuals to reclaim their sexual agency.

1

Social Dynamics and Connection

Group sex also taps into the human need for social connection and community. In many cultures, sexual encounters are often framed within the confines of intimate relationships. However, group scenarios can foster a sense of belonging and shared experience that transcends traditional boundaries. This is particularly appealing in the context of non-monogamous relationships, where individuals seek to explore their sexuality in a communal setting.

The dynamics of group sex can facilitate deeper connections between participants. The shared vulnerability inherent in these experiences can lead to heightened emotional intimacy and camaraderie. In this way, group sex acts as a catalyst for exploring not only physical pleasure but also emotional bonds, creating a unique interplay between eroticism and connection.

Biological Underpinnings

From a biological perspective, the allure of group sex can be linked to evolutionary theories surrounding reproductive strategies. The *dual mating strategy* suggests that individuals may be biologically predisposed to seek multiple partners to maximize reproductive success. This is particularly evident in women, who may experience heightened sexual arousal in group settings due to the presence of multiple potential mates.

Moreover, the release of hormones such as oxytocin during sexual encounters can enhance feelings of bonding and pleasure. In group scenarios, the collective experience may amplify these physiological responses, leading to heightened arousal and satisfaction. This biological framework helps explain why group sex can be such a compelling fantasy: it taps into primal instincts while simultaneously providing an avenue for exploration and pleasure.

Cultural Narratives and Media Influence

Cultural narratives and media representations also play a crucial role in shaping perceptions of group sex. Popular culture often glorifies group encounters, portraying them as adventurous and liberating experiences. This representation can create a sense of aspiration, encouraging individuals to explore their fantasies and desires.

However, it is essential to approach these portrayals critically. While media can normalize and validate group sex as a fantasy, it may also perpetuate unrealistic expectations and stereotypes. Engaging in group sex is not merely a series of sexual acts; it requires communication, consent, and emotional intelligence.

Understanding the distinction between fantasy and reality is crucial for navigating these experiences safely and consensually.

Conclusion

In summary, the popularity of group sex as a fantasy is rooted in a complex interplay of psychological, social, biological, and cultural factors. The thrill of the taboo, the desire for connection, biological instincts, and cultural narratives converge to create an enticing allure. As individuals explore these fantasies, it is vital to approach group encounters with a focus on consent, communication, and emotional well-being. By doing so, participants can fully embrace the potential for pleasure and connection that group sex offers, transforming a taboo into a celebration of sexual freedom and exploration.

Dispelling Myths: Addressing Concerns and Misconceptions

Group sexual encounters often come with a variety of myths and misconceptions that can create anxiety or deter individuals from exploring these experiences. In this section, we will address some of the most common myths surrounding group sex, providing clarity and understanding to empower readers in their journey toward pleasurable group experiences.

Myth 1: Group Sex is Only for the Sexually Promiscuous

One of the most pervasive myths is that only sexually promiscuous individuals engage in group sex. This stereotype can lead to feelings of shame or judgment for those who are curious about or interested in group encounters. However, the reality is that people from all walks of life, regardless of their sexual history, may seek out group experiences for various reasons, including exploration, connection, and pleasure. A study by [?] found that motivations for group sex included a desire for novelty, enhanced intimacy, and the opportunity to fulfill fantasies, rather than promiscuity.

Myth 2: Group Sex is Chaotic and Lacks Intimacy

Another common misconception is that group sex is chaotic and devoid of intimacy. This myth can stem from portrayals in media that emphasize wild, uninhibited behavior. In contrast, many individuals report that group encounters can foster deep connections and intimacy, as they often require heightened communication, trust, and vulnerability. Establishing clear boundaries and engaging in open discussions about desires can enhance emotional intimacy, allowing participants to feel more connected to one another.

Myth 3: Jealousy is Inevitable in Group Scenarios

Many people fear that jealousy is an unavoidable part of group sex. While it is true that jealousy can arise, it is not a foregone conclusion. Effective communication and setting clear expectations can significantly mitigate feelings of jealousy. For instance, utilizing techniques like *pre-play discussions* allows participants to express their feelings and establish agreements about how they will navigate interactions. Research by [?] indicates that partners who openly communicate their feelings and insecurities prior to engaging in group sex are better equipped to handle jealousy when it arises.

Myth 4: Group Sex is Only for Young People

The belief that group sex is exclusively for the young is another misconception that can deter individuals of all ages from exploring their sexuality. In reality, people of all ages engage in group encounters. A survey conducted by [?] revealed that individuals aged 40 and older reported enjoying group sex experiences, often citing increased confidence and self-awareness as factors that enhanced their enjoyment.

Myth 5: You Must Be an Expert to Participate

Many individuals shy away from group sex due to the belief that they must be highly experienced or skilled. This myth can create unnecessary pressure and inhibit exploration. The truth is that everyone starts somewhere, and group encounters can be an opportunity for mutual learning and discovery. Participants can engage in shared experiences, exploring pleasure together and developing skills in a supportive environment.

Myth 6: Group Sex is Unsafe

Concerns about safety in group sexual encounters are valid, but they are often based on misconceptions. While it is crucial to prioritize safety, many group scenarios are structured around consent, communication, and health practices. Establishing a culture of consent and utilizing safe sex practices, such as regular STI testing and the use of barriers, can create a safer environment. According to [?], groups that prioritize open discussions about health and consent report higher levels of satisfaction and lower instances of negative experiences.

Myth 7: Group Sex is Only About Physical Pleasure

Lastly, the idea that group sex is solely about physical pleasure overlooks the emotional and psychological aspects of these encounters. While physical pleasure is certainly a component, many participants find that group sex can enhance emotional intimacy, foster connections, and encourage personal growth. Engaging in group play can lead to increased self-awareness and a deeper understanding of one's desires and boundaries. A study by [?] highlighted that participants often reported a greater sense of community and connection after group encounters, emphasizing the multifaceted nature of these experiences.

Conclusion

Dispelling these myths is essential for creating a more inclusive and understanding perspective on group sexual encounters. By addressing concerns and misconceptions, individuals can approach group sex with confidence, clarity, and a sense of empowerment. The key to enjoying group scenarios lies in open communication, mutual consent, and a commitment to creating a safe and pleasurable environment for all participants. Embracing the diversity of experiences and motivations can lead to fulfilling and enriching sexual encounters, ultimately enhancing one's sexual journey.

Benefits of Group Sexual Encounters: Physiological and Emotional

Group sexual encounters offer a unique landscape for exploration, connection, and pleasure. Understanding the physiological and emotional benefits of these experiences can empower individuals to engage in them mindfully and joyfully.

Physiological Benefits

Engaging in group sexual encounters can have several physiological benefits that enhance overall sexual health and well-being.

1. **Enhanced Arousal and Orgasm Potential** Group settings often amplify arousal through a phenomenon known as *social facilitation*. This refers to the increased motivation and performance that can occur in the presence of others. The excitement of being watched or participating in a shared experience can lead to heightened sexual responses. Research indicates that the presence of multiple

partners can stimulate the release of hormones such as dopamine and oxytocin, enhancing pleasure and orgasm intensity.

$$\text{Arousal} \propto \text{Presence of Others} \cdot \text{Hormonal Release} \qquad (1)$$

2. Exploration of Varied Sexual Techniques Group encounters provide an opportunity to explore diverse sexual techniques and preferences. Participants can learn from each other, experimenting with different forms of touch, stimulation, and positions. This exchange of knowledge can lead to improved sexual skills and increased satisfaction. For instance, observing how a partner responds to certain touches can inform one's own approach, fostering a more responsive and fulfilling sexual experience.

3. Physical Health Benefits Engaging in sexual activity has been linked to numerous health benefits, including improved cardiovascular health, enhanced immune function, and reduced stress levels. Group encounters, with their often heightened levels of physical activity, can contribute to these benefits. According to the American Heart Association, regular sexual activity can be as effective as moderate exercise in promoting heart health.

$$\text{Health Benefits} = f(\text{Frequency of Sexual Activity, Intensity}) \qquad (2)$$

Emotional Benefits

Beyond the physiological aspects, group sexual encounters can offer significant emotional benefits that contribute to personal growth and relational dynamics.

1. Increased Emotional Connection Participating in group sexual encounters can foster deeper emotional connections among participants. The shared vulnerability and intimacy of such experiences can lead to stronger bonds. This sense of community and connection can enhance feelings of belonging and acceptance, which are crucial for emotional well-being.

2. Exploration of Identity and Desires Group settings can provide a safe space for individuals to explore their sexual identities and desires more freely. This exploration can lead to greater self-acceptance and understanding. For example, individuals who identify as non-binary or queer may find validation and affirmation in group encounters that embrace diverse sexual expressions.

3.   **Reducing Stigma and Shame**   Engaging in consensual group sexual encounters can help challenge societal taboos surrounding sexuality.   By participating in these experiences, individuals can reduce feelings of shame or guilt associated with their desires. This normalization can lead to healthier attitudes toward sexuality and enhance overall emotional health.

4. Coping with Jealousy and Insecurity   Group sexual encounters can also serve as a platform for addressing and overcoming feelings of jealousy and insecurity. By openly communicating and establishing trust within the group, participants can work through these emotions constructively. This process can lead to increased emotional resilience and a deeper understanding of personal boundaries and desires.

Conclusion

In summary, the physiological and emotional benefits of group sexual encounters are profound and multifaceted.   From enhancing arousal and exploring new techniques to fostering emotional connections and reducing stigma, these experiences can significantly enrich individuals' sexual lives. As with any sexual encounter, the key to maximizing these benefits lies in prioritizing consent, communication, and trust among all participants. Embracing the potential of group encounters can lead to a more fulfilling and empowered sexual journey.

Creating a Safe and Consensual Environment

Creating a safe and consensual environment is paramount in any sexual encounter, but it takes on even greater significance in group scenarios. The complexity of multiple individuals interacting can lead to a myriad of dynamics, requiring clear frameworks and practices to ensure that everyone involved feels secure, respected, and fully engaged in the experience.

Understanding Safety in Group Encounters

Safety in group sexual encounters encompasses both physical and emotional dimensions. Physically, it involves maintaining health standards, such as practicing safe sex and ensuring that all participants have consented to the activities planned. Emotionally, safety refers to creating an atmosphere where individuals feel free to express their desires, boundaries, and concerns without fear of judgment or coercion.

Physical Safety   Physical safety can be approached through a few key practices:

- **Health Checks:** Regular sexual health screenings should be a norm for all participants. Discussing STI status openly and honestly can help build trust and ensure that everyone is on the same page regarding risks.

- **Safe Sex Practices:** The use of condoms, dental dams, and other barriers is crucial in group settings. Not only do these practices protect against STIs, but they also foster a sense of security among participants.

- **Emergency Protocols:** Establishing a plan for emergencies is essential. This may involve designating a safe word or signal for anyone feeling uncomfortable, as well as having a first-aid kit readily available.

Emotional Safety   Emotional safety can be fostered through:

- **Open Communication:** Encouraging participants to express their feelings, boundaries, and preferences openly helps to cultivate a trusting environment. This can be facilitated through pre-play discussions or ice-breaking activities.

- **Consent Culture:** Consent is not a one-time agreement but an ongoing dialogue. Continuous check-ins during the encounter can help ensure that everyone remains comfortable and enthusiastic about their participation.

- **Aftercare:** Providing emotional support and aftercare post-encounter is vital. This may include cuddling, discussing the experience, or simply checking in on each other's emotional state.

Establishing Clear Boundaries

Setting boundaries is a critical component of any sexual encounter, particularly in group scenarios where various dynamics can come into play. Each participant should feel empowered to articulate their limits, and these boundaries must be respected by all involved.

Negotiating Boundaries   When negotiating boundaries, consider the following:

- **Personal Reflection:** Encourage participants to reflect on their own limits prior to the encounter. This self-awareness can help individuals articulate their needs clearly.

- **Group Discussions:** Facilitate a group discussion where everyone can share their boundaries. This not only fosters a sense of community but also ensures that everyone is aware of each other's limits.

- **Written Agreements:** In some cases, having a written agreement can help clarify and solidify boundaries. This can be particularly useful in larger groups or more complex scenarios.

Creating a Culture of Consent

A culture of consent is foundational to creating a safe environment in group sexual encounters. Consent should be informed, enthusiastic, and revocable at any time.

Informed Consent   Informed consent means that all participants understand what they are consenting to. This involves:

- **Full Disclosure:** Participants should provide full disclosure about their intentions and desires for the encounter. This includes discussing any activities that will take place and any specific preferences or limits.

- **Understanding Risks:** Participants should be aware of any physical or emotional risks involved in the activities they are consenting to. This allows for informed decision-making.

Enthusiastic Consent   Enthusiastic consent is a step beyond basic consent; it emphasizes the importance of participants being genuinely excited about engaging in the activities. This can be fostered by:

- **Encouraging Enthusiasm:** Create an environment where participants feel comfortable expressing their excitement and desires. This may involve playful conversations or activities that ignite passion and enthusiasm.

- **Checking In:** Regularly check in with participants during the encounter to ensure that everyone is still feeling enthusiastic and engaged.

Revocable Consent   Revocable consent acknowledges that individuals can change their minds at any point during the encounter. This principle can be reinforced by:

- **Safe Words:** Establishing a safe word or signal that any participant can use to pause or stop the encounter ensures that everyone knows they have the power to withdraw consent at any time.

+ **Creating a No-Pressure Environment:** Encourage participants to voice their feelings without fear of pressure or repercussions. This can help foster a more relaxed atmosphere where everyone feels safe to express their needs.

Addressing Power Dynamics

In group scenarios, power dynamics can become complex, particularly if there are differences in experience, status, or authority among participants. Addressing these dynamics is crucial to maintaining a safe and consensual environment.

Recognizing Power Imbalances   Participants should be encouraged to recognize and discuss any power imbalances that may exist. This can involve:

+ **Open Dialogue:** Create space for conversations about power dynamics and how they may affect individual experiences during the encounter.

+ **Empowering Voices:** Ensure that all participants feel empowered to speak up and share their perspectives, regardless of their perceived status within the group.

Creating Equitable Dynamics   To foster equitable dynamics:

+ **Encouraging Shared Leadership:** Rather than having a single leader or organizer, encourage shared leadership among participants to create a more balanced environment.

+ **Facilitating Group Decision-Making:**   Involve all participants in decision-making processes regarding activities and boundaries, ensuring that everyone's voice is heard and valued.

Conclusion

Creating a safe and consensual environment is not just a prerequisite for group sexual encounters; it is the foundation upon which pleasurable experiences are built. By prioritizing physical and emotional safety, establishing clear boundaries, fostering a culture of consent, and addressing power dynamics, participants can engage fully and joyfully in their shared experiences. Remember, the goal is not merely to avoid harm but to cultivate an atmosphere where everyone can thrive, explore, and revel in the pleasure of connection.

Consent, Boundaries, and Communication in Group Scenarios

In the realm of group sexual encounters, the principles of consent, boundaries, and effective communication are paramount. These elements not only ensure a safe and pleasurable experience but also cultivate an environment of trust and respect among participants. This section delves into the intricacies of these concepts, providing a framework to navigate the complexities of group dynamics.

Understanding Consent

Consent is an ongoing, affirmative agreement to engage in sexual activity. In group scenarios, it becomes even more critical due to the multiple participants involved. Each individual must feel empowered to voice their desires and limits. Consent can be visualized through the following equation:

$$\text{Consent} = \text{Informed} + \text{Freely Given} + \text{Reversible} + \text{Enthusiastic} \qquad (3)$$

- **Informed:** All parties must have a clear understanding of what the encounter entails.

- **Freely Given:** Consent should not be coerced or manipulated; it must come from a place of genuine desire.

- **Reversible:** Anyone can change their mind at any time, and this decision must be respected.

- **Enthusiastic:** Consent should be enthusiastic, indicating a genuine eagerness to participate.

Establishing Boundaries

Boundaries are personal limits that define what individuals are comfortable with in a sexual context. In group scenarios, discussing boundaries before engaging in sexual activities is essential. This can be facilitated through a pre-play discussion where participants share their limits, preferences, and any hard or soft boundaries they may have.

- **Hard Limits:** Activities that a participant is not willing to engage in under any circumstances (e.g., certain sexual acts, types of touch).

+ **Soft Limits:** Activities that may be acceptable under specific conditions or with certain partners but are not universally acceptable.

For example, one participant may have a hard limit against anal play, while another may have a soft limit that could be negotiated based on trust and comfort levels.

Effective Communication Strategies

Effective communication is the backbone of successful group sexual encounters. Here are several strategies to enhance communication:

+ **Use of Clear Language:** Avoid ambiguous terms; be specific about what you mean. Instead of saying, "I'm okay with that," clarify with "I would enjoy that."

+ **Active Listening:** Pay attention to what others are saying without planning your response while they speak. Reflect back what you hear to ensure understanding.

+ **Nonverbal Cues:** Be aware of body language, both your own and that of others. Nonverbal signals can often communicate discomfort or enthusiasm more than words.

Addressing Jealousy and Insecurity

Jealousy and insecurity can arise in group scenarios, particularly if individuals feel threatened by the attention others receive. It is vital to address these feelings openly. A simple check-in, such as asking, "How is everyone feeling about the dynamics right now?" can provide a platform for expressing concerns and reinforcing trust.

Establishing Consent Protocols

In group settings, establishing clear consent protocols can prevent misunderstandings. This may include:

+ **Consent Check-Ins:** Regularly pause during the encounter to ask if everyone is still comfortable and consenting to the activities taking place.

+ **Safe Words:** Agree on safe words that any participant can use to pause or stop the activity. This ensures that everyone has a tool for asserting their boundaries.

Navigating Group Dynamics

Understanding the dynamics of the group is crucial. Each participant brings their own experiences, desires, and boundaries. It is essential to create a space where everyone feels empowered to express themselves.

- **Group Agreements:** Before engaging, establish group agreements that outline how participants will communicate and respect each other's boundaries.

- **Role Assignments:** In some scenarios, assigning roles (such as a facilitator) can help manage the dynamics and ensure that all voices are heard.

Conclusion

Navigating consent, boundaries, and communication in group sexual encounters is not merely a checklist but a continuous practice of respect and awareness. By fostering an environment where everyone feels safe to express themselves, participants can enhance their collective experience, leading to deeper connections and greater pleasure. Remember, the journey of exploration in group dynamics is as much about personal empowerment as it is about shared enjoyment.

In summary, the integration of these principles creates a foundation for fulfilling and consensual group sexual encounters, leading to richer experiences for all involved. Embrace the power of communication, respect the boundaries set forth, and prioritize consent to ride the waves of pleasure together.

Building Trust and Establishing Rules for Group Play

Building trust and establishing rules are foundational elements for a successful and enjoyable group sexual encounter. Trust is the bedrock of any intimate relationship, and in group scenarios, it becomes even more critical due to the complexities of multiple partners and interactions. This section will explore how to cultivate trust and create a framework of rules that enhance safety, pleasure, and connection.

The Importance of Trust in Group Dynamics

Trust allows individuals to feel safe and secure in expressing their desires, boundaries, and vulnerabilities. In a group setting, where multiple people are engaging in sexual activities, the level of trust can significantly impact the experience. When trust is present, participants are more likely to communicate openly, engage in shared fantasies, and explore their sexuality without fear of judgment or harm.

Theoretical Framework   According to social penetration theory, intimacy develops through a gradual process of self-disclosure and vulnerability. In group sexual encounters, this theory underscores the importance of establishing trust before engaging in sexual activities. The more individuals share about their desires, boundaries, and experiences, the deeper the trust can grow, leading to more fulfilling encounters.

Problems Arising from Lack of Trust   Without trust, group dynamics can quickly deteriorate, leading to misunderstandings, discomfort, and even harm. Participants may feel anxious or insecure, which can inhibit their ability to enjoy the experience. Jealousy and competition can arise, particularly if individuals feel threatened by one another. Establishing trust mitigates these risks, allowing for a more enjoyable and liberated experience.

Establishing Rules for Group Play

Creating a set of rules is essential to ensure that everyone involved feels respected and safe. These rules should be established collaboratively and revisited regularly to adapt to the evolving dynamics of the group.

Key Rules to Consider

- **Consent is Paramount:** Every participant must give enthusiastic consent before engaging in any activity. Consent should be ongoing, meaning that anyone can withdraw their consent at any time.

- **Clear Communication:** Encourage open dialogue about desires, boundaries, and limits. Establish a safe word or signal that anyone can use to pause or stop the activity if they feel uncomfortable.

- **Respect Personal Boundaries:** Each participant should communicate their boundaries clearly, and these should be respected without question. This includes physical, emotional, and sexual boundaries.

- **Safety Practices:** Discuss and agree on safe sex practices, including the use of protection and regular STI testing. Establish protocols for emergencies or unexpected situations.

+ **Aftercare:** Plan for aftercare needs, as emotional and physical support is often required after intense sexual experiences. Discuss what aftercare looks like for each participant.

+ **Limit Group Size:** Depending on the comfort levels of participants, it may be beneficial to limit the number of people involved in the encounter to facilitate intimacy and connection.

Examples of Rule Establishment   Consider a scenario where a group of four individuals is preparing for a sexual encounter. Before engaging, they gather to discuss their desires and boundaries. Each person shares what they are comfortable with, such as specific activities they enjoy or limits they have. They agree on a safe word, "Pineapple," which anyone can use if they feel uncomfortable. By having this conversation before the encounter, they establish a foundation of trust and respect.

Building Trust Through Shared Experiences

Engaging in activities that foster connection outside of sexual contexts can also build trust. Group bonding experiences, such as sharing personal stories or engaging in non-sexual intimacy, can enhance feelings of safety and trust.

Techniques for Building Trust

+ **Icebreakers:** Use icebreaker games to help participants get to know each other better before engaging in sexual activities. This can create a sense of camaraderie and ease.

+ **Group Activities:** Engage in non-sexual activities, such as cooking together or participating in a group meditation. These experiences can foster connection and trust among participants.

+ **Active Listening:** Encourage participants to practice active listening during discussions about boundaries and desires. This builds respect and understanding, which are crucial for trust.

Conclusion   Building trust and establishing rules are essential components of successful group sexual encounters. By fostering an environment of safety, respect, and open communication, participants can explore their desires more freely and enjoyably. As the group dynamics evolve, revisiting and adjusting these rules will ensure that trust remains strong and that every participant feels valued and safe.

Embracing these principles will not only enhance the pleasure of the experience but also contribute to the emotional well-being of all involved.

Exploring Power Dynamics in Group Sexual Encounters

Power dynamics play a crucial role in shaping the experiences and outcomes of group sexual encounters. Understanding these dynamics can enhance pleasure, foster trust, and create a more fulfilling environment for all participants. This section delves into the complexities of power dynamics, offering insights into their implications, challenges, and potential benefits in group scenarios.

Understanding Power Dynamics

Power dynamics refer to the ways in which power is negotiated, expressed, and experienced between individuals in a given context. In group sexual encounters, these dynamics can manifest in various forms, including:

- **Hierarchical Power:** This involves established roles or statuses among participants, such as dominant/submissive relationships or variations in sexual experience and confidence.

- **Social Power:** Participants may hold different levels of social power based on factors like age, attractiveness, or charisma, which can influence interactions and sexual dynamics.

- **Emotional Power:** Emotional intelligence and the ability to navigate feelings can create power imbalances, affecting how individuals communicate their desires and boundaries.

- **Physical Power:** The physical attributes of individuals, such as strength or size, can also influence dynamics, especially in more physically engaging scenarios.

Understanding these forms of power is essential for fostering a healthy and consensual group sexual experience.

Theoretical Frameworks

Several theoretical frameworks can help elucidate the complexities of power dynamics in sexual encounters:

- **Foucault's Theory of Power:** Michel Foucault posits that power is not merely held but is relational and pervasive. In group sexual encounters, power is fluid and can shift between participants based on context, consent, and interaction.

- **Social Exchange Theory:** This theory suggests that relationships are formed through a cost-benefit analysis. In group scenarios, individuals may weigh their desires against potential risks, affecting their willingness to engage and their level of comfort.

- **Intersectionality:** This framework emphasizes the interconnected nature of social categorizations such as race, gender, and class, and how they create overlapping systems of discrimination or disadvantage. In group sex, recognizing intersectionality can help participants understand how their identities influence power dynamics.

Challenges in Navigating Power Dynamics

While exploring power dynamics can enhance experiences, it also presents challenges:

- **Miscommunication:** Power imbalances can lead to misunderstandings about consent and boundaries. Clear communication is vital to ensure that all participants feel safe and respected.

- **Jealousy and Insecurity:** Participants may grapple with feelings of jealousy or insecurity, especially if they perceive others as having more power or desirability. Addressing these feelings openly can mitigate tension.

- **Consent and Coercion:** The complexity of power dynamics raises concerns about the authenticity of consent. Participants must be vigilant to ensure that consent is freely given and that no one feels coerced into participating in activities they are uncomfortable with.

Navigating Power Dynamics for Enhanced Pleasure

To navigate power dynamics effectively and enhance pleasure in group encounters, consider the following strategies:

- **Establish Clear Communication:** Before engaging in group play, discuss desires, boundaries, and expectations openly. This helps create a shared understanding and fosters trust among participants.

+ **Negotiate Roles:** Participants can negotiate roles that align with their desires and comfort levels, whether that involves taking on a dominant or submissive role or simply participating as equals.

+ **Practice Active Listening:** Encourage participants to express their needs and desires, and practice active listening to ensure everyone feels heard and validated.

+ **Utilize Safe Words:** Establishing safe words can provide a mechanism for participants to communicate discomfort or a desire to pause or stop an activity, reinforcing the importance of consent.

+ **Encourage Reflection:** After the encounter, engage in a debriefing session where participants can share their experiences, feelings, and any concerns. This practice promotes emotional intimacy and helps address any lingering power dynamics.

Examples of Power Dynamics in Group Scenarios

To illustrate the impact of power dynamics in group sexual encounters, consider the following examples:

+ **The Dominant/Submissive Dynamic:** In a BDSM-oriented group encounter, participants may clearly define their roles as dominants or submissives. This dynamic can enhance pleasure for those who thrive in structured power exchanges, provided that consent and communication are prioritized.

+ **The Experienced vs. Inexperienced Dynamic:** In a group where some participants have more sexual experience than others, the more experienced individuals may inadvertently take control of the encounter. This can lead to feelings of inadequacy for less experienced participants unless efforts are made to ensure inclusivity and equal participation.

+ **The Gender Dynamic:** Gender roles can influence power dynamics in group encounters. For instance, societal norms may lead to male participants feeling entitled to assert dominance, while female participants may feel pressured to be submissive. Challenging these norms through open dialogue can create a more equitable environment.

Conclusion

Exploring power dynamics in group sexual encounters is essential for creating a safe, consensual, and pleasurable experience for all participants. By understanding the various forms of power, addressing challenges, and implementing strategies for effective navigation, individuals can enhance their experiences and foster deeper connections. Ultimately, embracing the complexities of power dynamics can lead to more fulfilling and empowering group sexual encounters, allowing everyone to ride the wave of pleasure together.

Overcoming Jealousy and Insecurity in Group Settings

Jealousy and insecurity can be significant barriers to enjoying the full potential of group sexual encounters. These emotions can manifest in various ways, often leading to misunderstandings and conflicts that detract from the overall experience. Understanding the roots of these feelings and developing strategies to address them is essential for fostering a positive and pleasurable environment.

Understanding Jealousy and Insecurity

Jealousy is a complex emotion that can arise from the fear of losing something valuable, whether it be a partner's affection, attention, or sexual interest. In the context of group sex, this fear can be amplified by the presence of multiple partners, each vying for attention and connection. Insecurity, on the other hand, often stems from a lack of self-confidence or self-worth, leading individuals to question their desirability or value in the eyes of their partners.

The psychological underpinnings of jealousy can be explained through the lens of attachment theory. According to Bowlby (1969), our early relationships with caregivers shape our attachment styles, which influence how we perceive and react to intimacy in adulthood. Those with anxious attachment styles may be particularly prone to jealousy, fearing abandonment or unreciprocated affection in group settings.

Common Triggers of Jealousy and Insecurity

Several factors can trigger feelings of jealousy and insecurity during group sexual encounters:

+ **Comparison with Others:** Individuals may compare themselves to other participants, questioning their attractiveness, skills, or desirability.

◆ **Fear of Abandonment:** The presence of multiple partners can evoke fears of being replaced or overlooked, leading to feelings of inadequacy.

◆ **Past Experiences:** Previous negative experiences in group settings or relationships can resurface, causing anxiety and insecurity.

◆ **Communication Gaps:** Lack of open communication about desires, boundaries, and feelings can exacerbate misunderstandings and insecurities.

Strategies for Overcoming Jealousy and Insecurity

To effectively manage jealousy and insecurity, individuals can implement several strategies that promote self-awareness, communication, and emotional resilience.

1. Build Self-Awareness Understanding one's triggers is the first step toward overcoming jealousy and insecurity. Keeping a journal to reflect on feelings before, during, and after group encounters can help individuals identify patterns and triggers. This self-reflection fosters a greater understanding of personal insecurities and allows for proactive management during group play.

2. Communicate Openly Establishing open lines of communication with partners is crucial. Discussing feelings of jealousy or insecurity can help normalize these emotions and create a supportive environment. For instance, partners can agree to check in with each other periodically throughout the encounter, providing reassurance and affirming their connection.

3. Establish Boundaries Setting clear boundaries can help mitigate feelings of jealousy. Discussing what is acceptable and what is not in advance allows all participants to feel secure in their choices. For example, agreeing on limits regarding physical touch or emotional connections can help individuals feel more comfortable and less threatened.

4. Practice Mindfulness Mindfulness techniques, such as deep breathing or grounding exercises, can help individuals stay present and manage anxiety during group encounters. By focusing on the sensations of the moment rather than potential insecurities, participants can enhance their pleasure and reduce feelings of jealousy.

5. Cultivate Self-Compassion Practicing self-compassion involves treating oneself with kindness and understanding rather than judgment. Reminding oneself that everyone has insecurities can help normalize these feelings and reduce their impact. Affirmations such as, "I am worthy of love and pleasure," can reinforce positive self-regard.

Example Scenario

Consider a situation where two partners, Alex and Jamie, are attending a group sexual encounter. Jamie feels a surge of jealousy when Alex begins to engage with another participant. Recognizing this emotion, Jamie takes a moment to breathe deeply and reflect on the source of their feelings. Instead of suppressing their emotions, Jamie communicates with Alex, expressing their discomfort and desire for reassurance.

In response, Alex reassures Jamie of their connection and commitment, emphasizing that their bond remains strong regardless of the group dynamics. This open communication not only alleviates Jamie's immediate feelings of jealousy but also strengthens the trust between them, enhancing their overall experience.

Conclusion

Overcoming jealousy and insecurity in group sexual encounters is an ongoing process that requires self-awareness, effective communication, and emotional resilience. By addressing these feelings head-on and employing practical strategies, individuals can create a more fulfilling and pleasurable environment for themselves and their partners. Embracing the complexity of human emotions and fostering open dialogue can transform potential obstacles into opportunities for deeper connection and enjoyment.

Bibliography

[1] Bowlby, J. (1969). *Attachment and Loss: Vol. 1. Attachment.* New York: Basic Books.

Navigating Different Types of Group Dynamics

Group sexual encounters can vary widely in their dynamics, influenced by the number of participants, their relationships with one another, and the specific environment in which the encounter takes place. Understanding these dynamics is crucial for fostering a pleasurable and consensual experience for everyone involved. This section explores various types of group dynamics, the challenges they present, and strategies for navigating them effectively.

Types of Group Dynamics

1. **Monogamous Couples with a Third Party:** This dynamic often involves a couple inviting a third person into their sexual experience. The primary relationship is the focus, and the third party may be viewed as an addition rather than an equal participant.

Challenges: - Jealousy may arise from either partner. - The third party may feel like an outsider, leading to discomfort.

Strategies: - Establish clear boundaries and communicate openly about desires and insecurities. - Engage in pre-play discussions to ensure everyone feels included and valued.

2. **Swinger Couples:** In this dynamic, couples engage in sexual activities with other couples or singles. The emphasis is often on shared enjoyment without emotional entanglements.

Challenges: - Misalignment of expectations regarding emotional involvement. - Potential for feelings of inadequacy or competition.

Strategies: - Discuss individual and shared expectations before engaging in group play. - Foster a supportive environment where partners feel safe to express their feelings.

3. **Polyamorous Groups:** These dynamics involve multiple partners who may have varying degrees of emotional and sexual relationships with one another.

Challenges: - Complex emotional landscapes can lead to misunderstandings and hurt feelings. - Navigating different relationship hierarchies can be challenging.

Strategies: - Regular check-ins and open communication are vital to maintaining emotional health. - Establishing agreements regarding time spent with each partner can help manage feelings of neglect.

4. **BDSM Groups:** In BDSM dynamics, power exchange is often central, with roles such as Dominant and submissive clearly defined.

Challenges: - Miscommunication about consent and limits can lead to emotional or physical harm. - The intensity of experiences may overwhelm some participants.

Strategies: - Use safe words and establish clear consent protocols before engaging in any activities. - Aftercare is essential to ensure emotional and physical well-being post-session.

5. **Casual Group Encounters:** These are often spontaneous and involve participants who may not know each other well.

Challenges: - Lack of established trust can lead to discomfort and anxiety. - Varying levels of experience and comfort with group sex can create imbalances.

Strategies: - Create a safe space for introductions and discussions about limits and preferences. - Encourage everyone to voice their comfort levels and boundaries before engaging in sexual activities.

Theoretical Frameworks for Understanding Group Dynamics

Understanding group dynamics in sexual encounters can be informed by several psychological theories:

1. **Social Exchange Theory:** This theory posits that individuals evaluate their relationships based on perceived benefits and costs. In group dynamics, participants may weigh the pleasure gained against potential emotional risks.

$$\text{Outcome} = \text{Benefits} - \text{Costs} \qquad (4)$$

Application: Encourage participants to openly discuss what they hope to gain from the encounter and any concerns they may have, creating a balanced perspective.

2. **Attachment Theory:** This framework suggests that individuals' attachment styles influence their relationships and interactions. In group sexual encounters,

understanding whether participants have secure, anxious, or avoidant attachment styles can help in navigating dynamics.

Application: Participants can reflect on their attachment styles and communicate these to foster understanding and minimize conflict.

3. **Group Cohesion Theory:** This theory emphasizes the importance of unity within a group. High cohesion can lead to more satisfying experiences, while low cohesion may result in discomfort and disconnect.

Application: Engage in bonding activities or discussions prior to sexual encounters to enhance group cohesion and trust.

Practical Examples of Navigating Dynamics

1. **Scenario:** A couple invites a friend to join them for a sexual encounter. During the encounter, the friend feels left out as the couple engages in intimate acts.

Solution: The couple should make a conscious effort to include their friend in the experience, perhaps by alternating attention or involving them in shared activities, ensuring everyone feels valued.

2. **Scenario:** In a polyamorous group, one partner feels neglected when their significant other spends more time with another partner.

Solution: Regularly scheduled group discussions can help address feelings of neglect and reinforce the importance of maintaining emotional connections across all relationships.

3. **Scenario:** A BDSM group is unsure about the limits of a new participant.

Solution: Conduct a pre-play meeting where everyone can discuss their boundaries, desires, and safe words, ensuring that all participants feel safe and informed.

Conclusion

Navigating different types of group dynamics requires awareness, communication, and a commitment to creating a safe and enjoyable experience for all participants. By understanding the unique challenges presented by various group structures and employing effective strategies, individuals can enhance their pleasure and deepen their connections during group sexual encounters. Emphasizing consent, trust, and open dialogue will lead to more fulfilling and empowering experiences, allowing everyone to ride the waves of pleasure together.

Understanding and Managing Expectations in Group Scenarios

Group sexual encounters can evoke a wide range of expectations, desires, and anxieties. Understanding and managing these expectations is crucial for fostering a positive and pleasurable experience for all participants. This section will delve into the theory behind expectations in sexual contexts, common problems that arise, and practical strategies for effectively managing expectations in group scenarios.

Theoretical Framework of Expectations

Expectations in sexual encounters are influenced by a variety of factors, including individual desires, societal norms, and previous experiences. According to the *Expectancy Theory*, individuals form expectations based on their beliefs about the outcomes of their actions. In sexual contexts, these expectations can shape how participants engage with one another and the overall dynamics of the encounter.

$$E = \sum_{i=1}^{n} P_i \cdot O_i \tag{5}$$

Where:

+ E = Expected outcome

+ P_i = Probability of outcome i

+ O_i = Value of outcome i

This equation illustrates that the overall expectation is a function of the perceived probability of various outcomes and their associated values. In group sexual encounters, participants may have differing expectations about pleasure, emotional connection, and the dynamics of interaction, which can lead to misunderstandings if not addressed.

Common Problems Arising from Expectations

1. **Misalignment of Expectations:** Participants may enter a group scenario with vastly different expectations regarding sexual activity, emotional involvement, and the level of intimacy. For example, one participant may expect a casual encounter focused solely on physical pleasure, while another may seek emotional connection and intimacy. This misalignment can lead to disappointment, frustration, and potential conflict.

2. **Fear of Judgment:** Individuals may feel pressure to conform to perceived norms or expectations within the group. This fear can inhibit authentic expression of desires and boundaries, leading to a less satisfying experience. For instance, a participant might feel compelled to engage in activities they are uncomfortable with to avoid judgment from others.

3. **Overwhelm and Anxiety:** The dynamics of group scenarios can be overwhelming, particularly for newcomers. Anxiety about performance, acceptance, or the ability to connect with multiple partners can cloud judgment and hinder enjoyment. This anxiety can manifest physically, impacting arousal and overall satisfaction.

4. **Unrealistic Expectations:** Media portrayals of group sex often depict idealized scenarios that do not reflect the complexities of real-life experiences. Participants may enter with unrealistic expectations regarding pleasure, connection, and the ease of navigating group dynamics, leading to dissatisfaction.

Strategies for Managing Expectations

1. **Open Communication:** Establishing clear and open lines of communication before and during the encounter is essential. Participants should share their expectations, desires, and boundaries openly. This practice not only fosters trust but also ensures that everyone is on the same page. Consider using a group discussion or a written agreement to outline individual expectations.

2. **Setting Realistic Goals:** Encourage participants to set realistic and achievable goals for the encounter. This could involve focusing on enjoyment rather than specific outcomes, such as the number of orgasms achieved. By emphasizing the journey over the destination, participants can reduce pressure and enhance overall pleasure.

3. **Regular Check-Ins:** During the encounter, regular check-ins can help participants gauge each other's comfort levels and satisfaction. Simple questions like "How is everyone feeling?" or "Is there anything anyone wants to adjust?" can facilitate ongoing communication and ensure that everyone's needs are being met.

4. **Cultivating Flexibility:** Encourage participants to remain flexible and open to spontaneity. Group dynamics can shift unexpectedly, and being adaptable can lead to unexpected pleasures and deeper connections. Emphasizing the importance of enjoying the moment rather than adhering strictly to preconceived notions can enhance the experience.

5. **Post-Encounter Reflection:** After the encounter, participants should engage in a reflective discussion about their experiences. This can help individuals process their feelings, address any unmet expectations, and reinforce positive aspects of the

encounter. This practice fosters emotional intimacy and allows for growth in future encounters.

Examples of Managing Expectations

Consider a scenario where a group of friends decides to explore a sexual encounter together. One participant, Alex, enters with the expectation of a fun, casual experience, while another, Jamie, hopes for a deeper emotional connection. Prior to the encounter, they engage in a discussion about their desires, ultimately agreeing to focus on mutual pleasure and enjoyment without the pressure of emotional intimacy.

During the encounter, Alex checks in with Jamie, asking if they are comfortable with the current activities. Jamie expresses a desire for more intimate touch, and Alex is open to adapting their approach. This open communication allows both participants to feel heard and respected, resulting in a more satisfying experience for both.

In another example, a group of individuals meets through an online platform for a sexual encounter. Beforehand, they establish a group chat to discuss boundaries, preferences, and expectations. This proactive approach helps participants feel more comfortable and reduces anxiety, leading to a more enjoyable and fulfilling experience.

Conclusion

Understanding and managing expectations in group sexual scenarios is vital for creating a positive and pleasurable experience for all participants. By fostering open communication, setting realistic goals, and cultivating flexibility, individuals can navigate the complexities of group dynamics effectively. Engaging in reflective practices post-encounter further enhances emotional intimacy and personal growth, paving the way for more fulfilling group sexual experiences in the future.

Preparing for Pleasure: Physical and Mental Preparations

Self-Exploration and Self-Knowledge

Understanding Your Own Sexual Preferences and Limitations

Understanding your sexual preferences and limitations is a fundamental step towards maximizing pleasure in group sexual encounters. This self-knowledge not only enhances your own experience but also contributes to the overall dynamics of the group, fostering a respectful and pleasurable environment for all participants.

The Importance of Self-Discovery

Self-discovery is a journey that involves exploring your desires, boundaries, and what brings you pleasure. According to sex educator Emily Nagoski, understanding your own sexuality is crucial for sexual well-being. This process can be broken down into several components:

- **Desires:** What do you want to experience? This could range from specific activities to emotional connections.

- **Boundaries:** What are your limits? Knowing what you are not comfortable with is just as important as knowing what you enjoy.

- **Triggers:** Are there specific situations or actions that cause discomfort or anxiety? Identifying these can help you navigate group dynamics more effectively.

Methods for Self-Exploration

1. **Journaling:** Writing about your sexual experiences, fantasies, and feelings can help clarify your preferences. Use prompts like "What excites me?" or "What makes me uncomfortable?" to guide your reflections.

2. **Solo Exploration:** Engaging in self-pleasure can provide insights into your body's responses. Experiment with different techniques, speeds, and types of stimulation to discover what feels best for you.

3. **Mindfulness Practices:** Techniques such as meditation and body scans can enhance your awareness of physical sensations and emotional responses, allowing you to better understand your preferences.

4. **Open Conversations:** Discussing your desires with trusted friends or partners can provide new perspectives and help you articulate your needs more clearly.

Recognizing Limitations

Understanding your limitations is equally essential. Limitations can stem from various sources, including:

- **Emotional Factors:** Past traumas or negative experiences can create barriers to certain activities. Acknowledging these feelings is the first step toward addressing them. - **Physical Limitations:** Health conditions or physical discomfort can impact your ability to engage in specific sexual activities. It's important to be aware of these and communicate them to your partners. - **Psychological Constraints:** Anxiety, fear of judgment, or performance pressure can hinder your enjoyment. Recognizing these mental blocks can help you find strategies to cope.

The Role of Communication

Once you have a clearer understanding of your preferences and limitations, effective communication becomes vital. Here are some strategies:

- **Use "I" Statements:** Express your needs using statements like "I feel…" or "I prefer…" to avoid sounding accusatory or demanding. - **Be Honest and Direct:** Clearly articulate what you are comfortable with and what you are not. This transparency builds trust within the group. - **Check-in Regularly:** During group encounters, take moments to assess how you and your partners are feeling. This can prevent misunderstandings and enhance enjoyment.

Practical Examples

Consider the following hypothetical scenarios that illustrate the importance of understanding your preferences and limitations:

1. **Scenario A:** You enjoy being touched but have a limit on the types of touch you find pleasurable. Before a group encounter, you communicate, "I love gentle caresses but find deep pressure uncomfortable." This clarity allows your partners to engage with you in a way that maximizes your pleasure.

2. **Scenario B:** You have a history of anxiety related to group settings. By acknowledging this limitation, you might choose to participate in smaller groups or establish a safe word that allows you to step back if you start to feel overwhelmed.

Conclusion

In conclusion, understanding your sexual preferences and limitations is a crucial foundation for engaging in group sexual encounters. This self-awareness not only enhances your personal pleasure but also contributes to a respectful and enjoyable environment for everyone involved. By engaging in self-exploration, recognizing your limitations, and practicing effective communication, you empower yourself and your partners to create fulfilling and pleasurable experiences together.

$$\text{Self-Awareness} = \text{Desires} + \text{Boundaries} + \text{Triggers} \qquad (6)$$

Embrace the journey of self-discovery, and remember that your pleasure matters—both in solo exploration and in the vibrant tapestry of group dynamics.

Rediscovering Your Erotic Self: Assessing Desires and Fantasies

In the journey towards maximizing pleasure in group sexual encounters, it is crucial to first embark on an intimate exploration of your own erotic self. This involves assessing your desires and fantasies, which can serve as the foundation for a fulfilling and empowered sexual experience. Understanding what arouses you, what excites you, and what holds you back can significantly enhance your engagement in group scenarios.

The Importance of Self-Assessment

Self-assessment is not merely a checklist; it is an ongoing dialogue with yourself about your sexual identity and preferences. According to sex educator Emily Nagoski, understanding your sexual well-being is essential for a fulfilling sexual life. This understanding can help you identify what you genuinely desire versus what societal norms or expectations might dictate.

$$D = P + E + C \tag{7}$$

Where:

- D = Desire

- P = Personal preferences

- E = Emotional connection

- C = Contextual factors (e.g., environment, partner dynamics)

This equation illustrates that desire is a complex interplay of personal preferences, emotional factors, and the context in which sexual experiences occur. By understanding these components, you can begin to articulate your desires more clearly.

Exploring Desires and Fantasies

1. **Journaling Your Fantasies**: One of the most effective ways to rediscover your erotic self is through journaling. Write down your fantasies without judgment. This exercise allows you to explore your imagination and recognize patterns in what excites you. For example, you might find that you are drawn to themes of power exchange, intimacy, or adventure.

2. **Engaging in Guided Visualization**: Use guided visualizations to explore different scenarios. This can help you uncover hidden desires and fantasies. Picture yourself in a group setting: What roles do you play? How do you feel? What sensations do you experience?

3. **Discussing with a Trusted Partner**: Open up conversations with a partner who you trust. Share your fantasies and desires in a safe space. This can lead to deeper intimacy and may help you articulate what you want in a group setting.

4. **Utilizing Resources**: Consider reading erotic literature or watching films that resonate with your interests. This exposure can help you identify what elements of sexuality excite you, providing insights into your own desires.

Addressing Emotional Blocks

While exploring your desires, it is also essential to address any emotional blocks or trauma that may hinder your sexual expression. Many individuals carry societal stigmas or personal experiences that can create barriers to fully embracing their erotic selves.

   - **Identifying Emotional Blocks**: Reflect on any past experiences that may have affected your sexual confidence. This could include negative messages about sex, past traumas, or feelings of shame. Acknowledge these feelings and consider discussing them with a therapist or a trusted confidant.

   - **Practicing Self-Compassion**: Be gentle with yourself as you navigate these feelings. Understand that it is okay to have complex emotions about your sexuality. Self-compassion allows you to accept your desires without judgment, fostering a healthier relationship with your erotic self.

Building Body Positivity and Confidence

Rediscovering your erotic self also involves cultivating body positivity and confidence. Recognizing your body as a source of pleasure is vital in group sexual encounters.

1. **Body Affirmations**: Engage in daily body affirmations that celebrate your uniqueness. Phrases like "My body is a vessel of pleasure" can help shift your mindset towards appreciation rather than criticism.

2. **Mindful Movement**: Explore forms of movement that connect you with your body, such as dance, yoga, or sensual movement classes. These practices can enhance your awareness of your body and its capabilities, fostering a sense of empowerment.

3. **Self-Exploration**: Engage in solo pleasure practices to deepen your connection with your body. Masturbation is a powerful tool for understanding your own pleasure and can help you articulate what feels good when you are with others.

Final Thoughts

Rediscovering your erotic self is a vital step in preparing for group sexual encounters. By assessing your desires and fantasies, addressing emotional blocks, and building body positivity, you create a solid foundation for engaging in pleasurable and fulfilling group experiences. Remember, the journey of self-discovery is ongoing, and embracing your erotic self can lead to a richer, more satisfying sexual life.

As you navigate this journey, keep in mind that your desires are valid, and exploring them is a powerful act of self-empowerment. Embrace the process, and allow yourself to ride the waves of your erotic exploration.

Identifying and Addressing Emotional Blocks or Trauma

In the journey toward maximizing pleasure in group sexual encounters, it is crucial to recognize and address any emotional blocks or trauma that may hinder one's ability to fully engage and enjoy the experience. Emotional blocks can manifest as anxiety, fear, shame, or guilt, and they often stem from past experiences or societal conditioning. Understanding and addressing these blocks is essential for fostering a fulfilling and pleasurable group sexual experience.

Understanding Emotional Blocks

Emotional blocks are psychological barriers that can prevent individuals from experiencing pleasure and intimacy. These blocks may arise from various sources, including:

- **Past Trauma:** Experiences of sexual abuse, assault, or negative sexual encounters can create deep-seated fears and anxieties that impede one's ability to engage in pleasurable activities.

- **Societal Conditioning:** Cultural narratives around sex, particularly those that stigmatize group sexual encounters, can lead to feelings of shame or guilt, creating an internal conflict that hinders enjoyment.

- **Fear of Judgment:** Concerns about how one may be perceived by others in a group setting can lead to self-consciousness and inhibit the ability to relax and enjoy the moment.

- **Attachment Styles:** Individuals with insecure attachment styles may struggle with trust and intimacy, affecting their ability to connect with partners in a group setting.

Recognizing these emotional blocks is the first step toward addressing them. Self-reflection and introspection can aid in identifying specific fears or anxieties that may surface in group sexual scenarios.

Addressing Emotional Blocks

Once emotional blocks are identified, it is essential to address them through various strategies that promote healing and self-acceptance:

+ **Therapeutic Support:** Engaging with a therapist who specializes in sexual health or trauma can provide a safe space to explore past experiences and work through emotional blocks. Techniques such as Cognitive Behavioral Therapy (CBT) can be particularly effective in reframing negative thought patterns related to sexuality.

+ **Mindfulness and Meditation:** Practicing mindfulness can help individuals stay present and reduce anxiety. Techniques such as focused breathing or body scans can promote relaxation and enhance awareness of bodily sensations, allowing for a more pleasurable experience.

+ **Journaling:** Writing about past experiences, feelings, and desires can facilitate emotional processing. Journaling can help individuals articulate their fears and identify patterns that may be holding them back from fully engaging in group sexual encounters.

+ **Open Communication:** Discussing emotional blocks with potential partners can foster understanding and support. Establishing a safe environment for sharing vulnerabilities can enhance trust and connection, making it easier to navigate any emotional challenges that arise during group play.

+ **Gradual Exposure:** For those with significant anxiety around group sexual encounters, gradual exposure can be beneficial. Starting with smaller, less intimidating group settings can help build confidence and reduce fear over time.

Examples of Emotional Blocks in Group Scenarios

Consider the following scenarios that illustrate common emotional blocks and potential strategies for addressing them:

+ **Scenario 1: Past Trauma** - A participant who experienced sexual abuse may find themselves feeling triggered by certain actions or dynamics within the group. They might experience panic or withdrawal during intimate moments. In this case, it is vital for the individual to communicate their boundaries clearly and seek therapeutic support to process their trauma.

Engaging in mindfulness practices before the encounter can also help ground them.

+ **Scenario 2: Societal Conditioning** - An individual may feel shame about participating in group sex due to cultural beliefs that stigmatize such encounters. This shame can manifest as self-doubt or anxiety. Addressing these feelings through education about consensual non-monogamy and open discussions with supportive partners can help reframe their perspective and foster a more positive outlook on their desires.

+ **Scenario 3: Fear of Judgment** - A participant may worry excessively about how they will be perceived by others in the group, leading to self-consciousness that detracts from their enjoyment. Practicing self-compassion and reminding themselves that everyone is there to explore pleasure can alleviate these feelings. Engaging in pre-play discussions about desires and boundaries can also create a more supportive environment.

+ **Scenario 4: Attachment Issues** - An individual with an anxious attachment style may feel insecure about their place within the group, fearing they will not be chosen or valued. Addressing these feelings through open communication with partners and establishing clear agreements about emotional support can help mitigate these insecurities.

Conclusion

Identifying and addressing emotional blocks or trauma is a vital step in enhancing pleasure during group sexual encounters. By fostering self-awareness, engaging in therapeutic practices, and maintaining open communication with partners, individuals can work toward overcoming these barriers. Ultimately, the goal is to create a safe and pleasurable environment where all participants can fully embrace their desires and explore the depths of their sexual experiences together.

By acknowledging and addressing emotional blocks, individuals can unlock their potential for pleasure, connection, and joy in the realm of group sexual encounters.

Cultivating Body Positivity and Confidence

In the realm of group sexual encounters, cultivating body positivity and confidence is essential for maximizing pleasure and enhancing the overall experience. Body positivity refers to the acceptance of one's body, regardless of its shape, size, or any perceived imperfections. Confidence, on the other hand, is the belief in one's abilities and worth. Together, these elements create a foundation for enjoyable and fulfilling sexual experiences.

Understanding Body Positivity

Body positivity is rooted in the idea that all bodies are worthy of love and respect. It challenges societal norms and unrealistic beauty standards that often lead individuals to feel inadequate or insecure about their bodies. According to the *Body Image and Sexuality* study by Tiggermann and Slater (2013), individuals with a positive body image are more likely to engage in sexual activities and report higher levels of sexual satisfaction.

$$\text{Body Positivity} = \frac{\text{Acceptance of Body}}{\text{Societal Standards}} \tag{8}$$

This equation illustrates that body positivity increases as acceptance of one's body rises, while societal standards exert less influence.

The Impact of Body Confidence on Sexual Experiences

Confidence in one's body can significantly influence sexual experiences, particularly in group settings where vulnerability may be heightened. Research by Murnen et al. (2003) indicates that individuals who feel good about their bodies are more likely to engage in open communication about desires and boundaries, ultimately leading to more satisfying encounters.

$$\text{Confidence} = \text{Self-Acceptance} + \text{Positive Affirmations} \tag{9}$$

This equation highlights that confidence can be bolstered through self-acceptance and positive affirmations, which reinforce a healthy self-image.

Common Barriers to Body Positivity and Confidence

Despite the benefits, many individuals face barriers that hinder their ability to cultivate body positivity and confidence:

+ **Negative Self-Talk:** Internal dialogues that criticize one's appearance can diminish self-esteem. Combatting this requires conscious effort to replace negative thoughts with positive affirmations.

+ **Comparison Culture:** Social media and societal expectations often lead to unhealthy comparisons. Recognizing that everyone has unique attributes can help mitigate these feelings.

+ **Past Experiences:** Trauma or negative experiences related to body image can create lasting impacts. Seeking therapy or support groups can aid in processing these feelings.

Strategies for Cultivating Body Positivity and Confidence

To overcome these barriers, individuals can adopt several strategies:

+ **Practice Mindfulness:** Mindfulness techniques can help individuals become more attuned to their bodies and foster a sense of appreciation. Engaging in body scans or guided meditations focusing on body acceptance can enhance this awareness.

+ **Affirmations and Positive Self-Talk:** Creating a list of affirmations that celebrate one's body can be a powerful tool. For example, repeating phrases such as "My body is strong and capable" or "I am worthy of pleasure" can shift mindset over time.

+ **Surround Yourself with Positivity:** Engaging with body-positive communities, whether online or in-person, can provide support and encouragement. Following body-positive influencers and participating in discussions can foster a more accepting environment.

+ **Celebrate Small Wins:** Acknowledging and celebrating small achievements related to body positivity can reinforce confidence. Whether it's wearing an outfit that makes you feel good or trying a new activity, these moments are vital.

Examples of Body Positivity in Group Scenarios

In group sexual encounters, body positivity can manifest in various ways:

+ **Compliments and Affirmations:** Participants can create an atmosphere of positivity by offering genuine compliments to one another, reinforcing the idea that all bodies are beautiful and deserving of pleasure.

+ **Inclusive Practices:** Organizing group encounters that celebrate diversity in body types can enhance comfort levels. For example, creating spaces where all body types are represented and appreciated can foster a sense of belonging.

+ **Body-Positive Activities:** Engaging in activities that promote body appreciation, such as group yoga or sensual dance, can help individuals connect with their bodies and enhance confidence.

Conclusion

Cultivating body positivity and confidence is not just a personal journey but a collective one, especially in the context of group sexual encounters. By embracing our bodies and fostering an environment of acceptance, we can enhance our experiences and maximize pleasure. Remember, every body is a beautiful body, and confidence is the key that unlocks the door to deeper connections and more fulfilling sexual experiences. As we ride the waves of pleasure together, let us celebrate the unique beauty each person brings to the experience.

Exploring Solo Pleasure and Masturbation Techniques

Masturbation is a fundamental aspect of sexual exploration that allows individuals to develop a deeper understanding of their own bodies, preferences, and desires. In the context of preparing for group sexual encounters, solo pleasure serves not only as a means of self-discovery but also as a vital tool for enhancing sexual confidence and performance.

The Importance of Solo Pleasure

Engaging in solo pleasure offers numerous benefits:

- **Self-Discovery:** Through masturbation, individuals can explore their bodies, discover erogenous zones, and learn what types of stimulation lead to pleasure. This self-knowledge can be invaluable when communicating desires and preferences in group settings.

- **Stress Relief:** Masturbation can serve as a healthy outlet for stress and anxiety, promoting relaxation and emotional well-being. This is particularly beneficial before entering the potentially vulnerable environment of group sex.

- **Enhanced Arousal:** Regular solo pleasure can help increase sensitivity and arousal levels, making it easier to reach orgasm during group encounters.

- **Skill Development:** Practicing different techniques during solo sessions can lead to improved sexual skills that can be shared with partners in group scenarios.

Masturbation Techniques

Understanding various masturbation techniques can empower individuals to maximize their pleasure. Here, we explore different approaches that can be tailored to personal preferences.

1. Manual Stimulation   Manual stimulation involves using the hands to stimulate the genitals. Key techniques include:

+ **The Basic Stroke:** For those with a clitoris, a gentle rubbing motion using the fingers can be effective. Experimenting with different pressures and speeds can lead to varied sensations.

+ **Varying Techniques:** Individuals can explore techniques such as circular motions, tapping, or even pinching to discover what feels best. For those with a penis, stroking along the shaft while varying grip strength can enhance pleasure.

2. Incorporating Lubrication   Lubricants can significantly enhance the experience of solo pleasure. The use of water-based, silicone-based, or oil-based lubricants can reduce friction and heighten sensations.

$$\text{Pleasure} = \text{Stimulation} + \text{Lubrication} + \text{Technique} \tag{10}$$

3. Using Sex Toys   Sex toys can add an exciting dimension to solo pleasure. Options include:

+ **Vibrators:** These can provide targeted stimulation to erogenous zones. Experimenting with different settings can help individuals find their optimal pleasure level.

+ **Dildos:** For those interested in penetration, dildos can be used to explore internal sensations, such as G-spot or prostate stimulation.

4. Exploring Fantasy and Visualization   Incorporating fantasy can enhance arousal during solo sessions. Visualization techniques might include:

+ **Erotic Literature:** Reading erotic stories or watching adult films can stimulate the imagination, making solo pleasure more engaging.

+ **Mindfulness Techniques:** Focusing on sensations and being present in the moment can enhance the experience. Techniques such as deep breathing or body scanning can help individuals connect more deeply with their pleasure.

Common Challenges and Solutions

While exploring solo pleasure, individuals may encounter challenges. Here are some common issues and potential solutions:

1. Performance Anxiety It's common for individuals to feel pressure to perform or achieve orgasm. Remember that the goal of solo pleasure is exploration, not necessarily climax. Techniques to alleviate anxiety include:

+ **Setting the Scene:** Creating a comfortable and private environment can help ease nerves.

+ **Practicing Self-Compassion:** Remind yourself that there is no right or wrong way to experience pleasure.

2. Emotional Blocks Past traumas or negative experiences can hinder the ability to enjoy solo pleasure. Techniques to address emotional blocks include:

+ **Journaling:** Writing about feelings related to sexuality can help process emotions and reduce anxiety.

+ **Seeking Professional Support:** Therapy or counseling can provide a safe space to explore and address deeper issues.

3. Boredom with Routine To keep solo pleasure exciting, individuals can:

+ **Change Techniques:** Regularly experimenting with new techniques or toys can reinvigorate the experience.

+ **Incorporate Role-Play:** Engaging in role-play scenarios during solo sessions can add an element of fun and creativity.

Conclusion

Exploring solo pleasure and masturbation techniques is an empowering journey that enhances sexual well-being and confidence. By understanding one's own body and preferences, individuals can approach group sexual encounters with greater self-assurance and a deeper connection to their own pleasure. Embrace this exploration as a vital part of your sexual journey, unlocking the potential for greater enjoyment in all aspects of your sexual life.

Techniques for Enhancing Arousal and Amplifying Sensations

Enhancing arousal and amplifying sensations are key components in maximizing pleasure during group sexual encounters. Understanding the intricacies of human sexuality can empower individuals to explore their desires more fully and to connect with others in profound and pleasurable ways. This section will delve into various techniques that can enhance arousal and amplify sensations, providing practical strategies for individuals looking to elevate their experiences in group settings.

1. The Role of Anticipation

Anticipation is a powerful aphrodisiac. The buildup of desire before physical intimacy can significantly enhance arousal. Techniques to cultivate anticipation include:

+ **Teasing and Flirting:** Engage in playful teasing, both verbally and physically. This can involve light touches, suggestive comments, or playful banter that builds sexual tension.

+ **Setting the Scene:** Create an erotic atmosphere with dim lighting, sensual music, and comfortable spaces that invite intimacy. The environment plays a crucial role in enhancing arousal.

+ **Delayed Gratification:** Practice delaying certain pleasures to increase desire. For example, engage in prolonged foreplay or take turns focusing on each other's pleasure without immediate climax.

2. Sensory Stimulation

The body is a canvas of sensations, and enhancing these can lead to heightened arousal. Consider the following techniques:

+ **Sensory Play:** Incorporate elements that stimulate the senses—such as feathers, ice, or warm oils—to explore different textures and temperatures on the skin. This can create a heightened awareness of touch and sensation.

+ **Blindfolding:** Removing the sense of sight can amplify other senses. Blindfolds can lead to heightened anticipation and sensitivity to touch, sound, and smell.

+ **Aromatherapy:** Utilize scents that are known to enhance sexual arousal, such as jasmine, ylang-ylang, or sandalwood. Scents can evoke emotional responses and enhance the overall experience.

3. Breathwork and Mindfulness

Breath is a powerful tool for enhancing arousal and connecting with oneself and partners. Techniques include:

+ **Deep Breathing:** Engage in deep, rhythmic breathing to increase oxygen flow and relaxation. This can enhance physical sensations and emotional connection during intimate moments.

+ **Mindfulness Practices:** Focus on being present in the moment. Mindfulness can enhance awareness of physical sensations and emotional responses, allowing for a deeper connection with oneself and others.

+ **Synchronizing Breath:** In a group setting, try synchronizing breaths with partners. This can create a shared energy and enhance the collective experience of arousal.

4. Exploring Erogenous Zones

Understanding and stimulating erogenous zones can lead to amplified sensations. Techniques include:

+ **Identifying Erogenous Zones:** Each individual has unique sensitive areas. Common erogenous zones include the neck, inner thighs, and lower back. Explore these areas through touch, kisses, or gentle bites.

+ **Varying Pressure and Speed:** Experiment with different pressures and speeds when touching erogenous zones. What feels good can vary greatly from person to person and even from moment to moment.

+ **Using Lubricants:** Incorporate lubricants to enhance sensations during touch. The right lubricant can reduce friction and increase pleasure, making every caress feel more intense.

5. Incorporating Toys and Props

Using sex toys and props can significantly enhance arousal and sensations. Consider the following:

+ **Vibrators and Dildos:** Introduce vibrators or dildos into group play to stimulate various erogenous zones. Different types of toys can provide unique sensations and enhance pleasure for all involved.

+ **Bondage Gear:** Incorporating elements of bondage, such as restraints or blindfolds, can heighten anticipation and arousal. The element of control can amplify sensations and create a thrilling dynamic.

+ **Temperature Play:** Use heated or chilled toys to explore temperature contrasts on the skin. This can create intense sensations that heighten arousal.

6. Communication and Feedback

Open communication is essential for enhancing arousal in group settings. Techniques include:

+ **Verbal Feedback:** Encourage partners to express what feels good and what doesn't. Verbalizing pleasure can enhance arousal and create a more connected experience.

+ **Non-Verbal Cues:** Pay attention to body language and non-verbal signals. Understanding and responding to these cues can enhance the overall experience.

+ **Setting Safe Words:** Establish safe words to ensure everyone feels comfortable and can communicate boundaries effectively. This fosters a safe environment for exploration.

7. The Power of Connection

Emotional and physical connection can significantly enhance arousal. Techniques include:

+ **Eye Contact:** Maintain eye contact with partners to create intimacy and connection. This can deepen emotional bonds and enhance physical pleasure.

+ **Touching and Cuddling:** Engage in non-sexual touching and cuddling to build intimacy. This can create a sense of safety and comfort that enhances arousal.

+ **Sharing Fantasies:** Discuss fantasies with partners to create a shared erotic narrative. This can enhance arousal and create a deeper connection between participants.

Conclusion

Enhancing arousal and amplifying sensations during group sexual encounters requires a combination of anticipation, sensory stimulation, mindfulness, and communication. By exploring these techniques, individuals can cultivate richer, more pleasurable experiences that deepen connections with themselves and their partners. Remember, the journey of sexual exploration is personal and unique; embrace it with an open heart and mind, and allow pleasure to guide the way.

Developing Mindfulness and Sensual Awareness

In the realm of sexual encounters, especially within group dynamics, the ability to be present and aware of one's own body and sensations is paramount. Mindfulness and sensual awareness enhance the quality of experiences, allowing individuals to fully engage with their own pleasure and that of their partners. This section explores the importance of these practices, the challenges individuals may face, and practical techniques to cultivate mindfulness and sensual awareness in group sexual scenarios.

The Importance of Mindfulness in Sexual Encounters

Mindfulness, defined as the practice of being fully present and engaged in the moment without judgment, can significantly impact sexual pleasure. Research in sexology indicates that individuals who practice mindfulness during sexual activities report higher levels of sexual satisfaction, enhanced arousal, and a greater capacity for experiencing orgasms. This phenomenon can be attributed to the following factors:

+ **Heightened Sensory Awareness:** Mindfulness encourages individuals to focus on their physical sensations, allowing them to experience pleasure more intensely. By tuning into the body, one can notice subtle changes in arousal and respond accordingly.

+ **Reduced Anxiety:** Mindfulness practices, such as meditation and deep breathing, can alleviate performance anxiety and distractions that often arise in group settings. This creates a more relaxed atmosphere conducive to pleasure.

+ **Enhanced Connection:** Being mindful allows individuals to connect more deeply with their partners. This connection fosters emotional intimacy, which can amplify physical pleasure.

Challenges to Mindfulness in Group Scenarios

While mindfulness can significantly enhance sexual experiences, several challenges may impede its practice in group encounters:

+ **Distractions:** In a group setting, external stimuli such as sounds, movements, and the presence of multiple partners can distract individuals from their own sensations.

+ **Self-Consciousness:** Concerns about body image, performance, or how one is perceived by others can lead to a lack of focus on personal pleasure.

+ **Emotional Turmoil:** Feelings of jealousy, insecurity, or anxiety about group dynamics can interfere with the ability to remain present and engaged.

Techniques for Cultivating Mindfulness and Sensual Awareness

To overcome these challenges and foster mindfulness and sensual awareness, individuals can employ several techniques:

1. **Breath Awareness** Focusing on the breath is a fundamental mindfulness practice. In group scenarios, individuals can use breath as an anchor to maintain presence. For example, participants can take a few deep breaths, inhaling through the nose and exhaling through the mouth, allowing themselves to feel the

sensations of the air entering and leaving their bodies. This practice can help ground individuals, making it easier to tune into their physical sensations.

2. Body Scan Meditation A body scan involves mentally scanning the body from head to toe, paying attention to areas of tension or pleasure. Practicing this technique before group encounters can enhance awareness of bodily sensations. During the encounter, individuals can periodically return to this practice, checking in with their bodies and noticing any changes in sensation.

3. Sensory Exploration Encouraging participants to engage in sensory exploration can heighten awareness. This can include focusing on different textures, temperatures, and sensations during foreplay. For instance, using silk scarves, ice cubes, or warm oils can stimulate the senses and create a heightened state of arousal, making it easier to remain present.

4. Mindful Touch Practicing mindful touch involves being fully present during physical contact with oneself or others. Participants can take turns exploring each other's bodies, focusing on the sensation of touch and the responses it elicits. This practice encourages communication about what feels good and fosters a deeper connection between partners.

5. Setting Intentions Before entering a group scenario, individuals can set intentions related to mindfulness and sensual awareness. For example, one might intend to remain present, explore sensations fully, or communicate openly with partners. This intention-setting can serve as a reminder throughout the encounter to return to a mindful state.

6. Engaging in Group Mindfulness Exercises Incorporating group mindfulness exercises, such as guided meditations or breath synchronization, can help establish a collective atmosphere of presence. This can be particularly effective in creating a safe space where all participants feel comfortable exploring their sensations together.

Practical Example: Mindfulness in Action

Consider a scenario where a group of individuals has gathered for a sexual encounter. Before engaging in any activities, they take a moment to sit in a circle, close their eyes, and focus on their breathing. After a few minutes, they engage in a body scan, allowing each participant to express what they feel in their bodies. This practice not only enhances individual awareness but also fosters a sense of shared experience.

As the encounter progresses, participants are encouraged to communicate openly about their sensations and desires. One partner might say, "I love it when you touch my back like that," while another might express their need for more gentle pressure. This open dialogue, grounded in mindfulness, allows for a more fulfilling and pleasurable experience for everyone involved.

Conclusion

Developing mindfulness and sensual awareness is a powerful tool for enhancing pleasure in group sexual encounters. By cultivating these practices, individuals can overcome distractions, reduce anxiety, and connect more deeply with themselves and their partners. The journey towards greater sexual fulfillment begins with the simple act of being present—an act that can transform not only individual experiences but also the collective energy of group play.

Maintaining Emotional Health and Well-being in Group Scenarios

Engaging in group sexual encounters can be exhilarating and liberating, but it also presents unique emotional challenges that require attention and care. Maintaining emotional health and well-being is essential for ensuring that all participants have a positive experience and feel safe and respected throughout the process. This section delves into strategies for nurturing emotional health before, during, and after group scenarios.

Understanding Emotional Dynamics

Group sexual encounters often involve a complex interplay of emotions, including excitement, vulnerability, jealousy, and connection. Understanding these dynamics is crucial for maintaining emotional well-being. Theories from psychology, such as *Attachment Theory*, suggest that our attachment styles can influence how we interact with others in intimate settings. Those with secure attachment styles may navigate group dynamics more easily, while those with anxious or avoidant styles may find themselves struggling with feelings of insecurity or isolation.

Anticipating Emotional Responses

Before participating in a group encounter, it's important to anticipate potential emotional responses. Common feelings may include:

+ **Excitement:** The thrill of new experiences can heighten arousal and connection.

+ **Jealousy:** Fears of inadequacy or exclusion may arise, particularly if one partner interacts closely with others.

+ **Vulnerability:** Exposing oneself emotionally and physically can lead to feelings of vulnerability.

+ **Connection:** Positive emotional bonds can develop, enhancing the overall experience.

Recognizing these emotions can help participants prepare mentally and emotionally, fostering a more enjoyable experience.

Communicating Needs and Boundaries

Effective communication is the cornerstone of emotional health in group scenarios. Participants should openly discuss their needs, boundaries, and any potential triggers that may arise during the encounter. This can include:

+ **Expressing Concerns:** Sharing fears or insecurities can create an environment of trust and support.

+ **Setting Boundaries:** Clearly defining personal limits helps prevent discomfort and emotional distress.

+ **Establishing Check-Ins:** Agreeing to periodic check-ins during the encounter allows participants to gauge emotional well-being and adjust as necessary.

Practicing Emotional Self-Care

Self-care practices are vital for maintaining emotional health in group settings. Consider the following strategies:

+ **Mindfulness Techniques:** Engaging in mindfulness exercises, such as deep breathing or meditation, can help ground participants and reduce anxiety.

+ **Journaling:** Writing about feelings before and after encounters can provide clarity and facilitate emotional processing.

+ **Self-Compassion:** Practicing self-compassion allows individuals to acknowledge their feelings without judgment, fostering emotional resilience.

Aftercare: Nurturing Emotional Recovery

Aftercare is a critical component of emotional health in group encounters. It involves providing support and care to one another after the experience, which can mitigate any negative feelings that arise. Effective aftercare practices include:

- **Cuddling and Physical Touch:** Engaging in gentle touch can promote feelings of safety and connection.

- **Discussing the Experience:** Sharing thoughts and feelings about the encounter can foster intimacy and understanding among participants.

- **Addressing Emotional Fallout:** If negative feelings arise, addressing them promptly through open communication helps prevent resentment or discomfort.

Recognizing Signs of Emotional Distress

Participants should be vigilant about recognizing signs of emotional distress in themselves and others. Common indicators may include:

- **Withdrawal:** A participant may become quiet or disengaged, signaling discomfort.

- **Irritability:** Increased irritability or frustration may indicate underlying emotional issues.

- **Physical Symptoms:** Stress can manifest physically, leading to symptoms like tension, headaches, or fatigue.

When signs of distress are recognized, it is important to address them with empathy and understanding, offering support or a break as needed.

Building a Supportive Community

Lastly, fostering a supportive community among group participants can enhance emotional well-being. This can involve:

- **Regular Group Meetings:** Establishing regular gatherings to discuss experiences and feelings can strengthen bonds and build trust.

- **Encouraging Open Dialogue:** Creating an environment where participants feel safe discussing their emotions promotes emotional health.

⁺ **Offering Peer Support:** Encouraging participants to support one another emotionally reinforces community and connection.

In conclusion, maintaining emotional health and well-being in group sexual encounters requires intentionality and care. By understanding emotional dynamics, communicating openly, practicing self-care, and fostering a supportive community, participants can enhance their experiences and navigate the complexities of group intimacy with confidence and joy.

Strengthening Intimacy and Connection with Partners

In the realm of group sexual encounters, cultivating intimacy and connection with partners is paramount. This section delves into the significance of emotional bonding and practical strategies to enhance intimacy, ensuring that every participant feels valued and connected.

Understanding Intimacy in Group Dynamics

Intimacy transcends mere physical interaction; it encompasses emotional, psychological, and even spiritual connections. According to [?], attachment theory posits that secure attachments foster trust and safety, which are crucial in group sexual settings. Intimacy can be understood through three primary dimensions:

⁺ **Emotional Intimacy:** Sharing feelings, thoughts, and vulnerabilities.

⁺ **Physical Intimacy:** Engaging in affectionate and sexual touch.

⁺ **Intellectual Intimacy:** Connecting through shared ideas and stimulating conversations.

Creating a strong foundation of intimacy can enhance the overall experience, allowing participants to explore their desires freely and confidently.

The Role of Communication

Effective communication is the bedrock of intimacy. In group scenarios, open dialogue about desires, boundaries, and feelings is essential. [?] emphasizes that couples who communicate effectively are more likely to maintain a healthy relationship. Here are some strategies to foster communication:

1. **Check-Ins:** Regularly ask partners how they feel about the experience. Simple questions like, "How is everyone feeling?" or "What do you need right now?" can open the floor for discussion.

2. **Expressing Gratitude:** Acknowledging and appreciating partners for their participation can strengthen bonds. Phrases like, "I loved how you touched me during that moment," can reinforce positive feelings.

3. **Active Listening:** Show genuine interest in what partners share. Reflect back what you hear to validate their feelings, which can create a deeper emotional connection.

Creating Shared Experiences

Shared experiences can significantly enhance intimacy. Engaging in activities that promote bonding before and after sexual encounters can help solidify connections. Here are some examples:

- **Group Activities:** Participating in activities like dancing, cooking, or playing games can break the ice and create a relaxed atmosphere.

- **Bonding Rituals:** Establishing rituals, such as a group hug before starting or a shared toast afterward, can create a sense of unity.

- **Collaborative Exploration:** Exploring fantasies or engaging in role-play scenarios together can deepen intimacy by fostering trust and vulnerability.

Navigating Vulnerability and Trust

Vulnerability is a double-edged sword; it can lead to deeper connections or potential hurt. In group settings, it's essential to navigate vulnerability with care. [?] suggests that vulnerability is the birthplace of innovation, creativity, and change. Here's how to approach vulnerability:

1. **Establish Trust:** Before engaging in group play, take time to build trust. This can be achieved through honest conversations about expectations and boundaries.

2. **Share Personal Stories:** Sharing personal experiences can foster a sense of vulnerability and encourage others to open up. This could include discussing past sexual experiences, fears, or desires.

3. **Create a Safe Space:** Ensure that everyone feels safe to express themselves without judgment. This can be reinforced by setting clear group agreements and consent protocols.

Addressing Emotional Needs

Recognizing and addressing emotional needs is vital in maintaining intimacy. Each partner may have unique emotional requirements that must be understood and respected. Here are some common emotional needs to consider:

+ **Affection:** Many people thrive on physical touch and affection. Regularly checking in to provide affectionate gestures can strengthen bonds.

+ **Validation:** Partners may need reassurance that their feelings and desires are valid. Acknowledging their emotions can foster a deeper connection.

+ **Security:** Providing a sense of safety and security is crucial. This can be achieved through clear communication and consistent behavior.

Practicing Aftercare

Aftercare is an essential practice that can significantly enhance intimacy post-encounter. It involves attending to the emotional and physical needs of all participants after a sexual experience. [?] highlights the importance of aftercare in maintaining emotional well-being. Here are some aftercare strategies:

+ **Cuddling and Physical Touch:** Engaging in affectionate touch after play can reinforce feelings of safety and connection.

+ **Emotional Check-Ins:** Discussing the experience and how everyone felt can help process emotions and reinforce bonds.

+ **Hydration and Nourishment:** Providing snacks and drinks can help participants feel cared for and appreciated.

Conclusion

Strengthening intimacy and connection with partners in group sexual encounters is a multifaceted process that involves effective communication, shared experiences, trust, and aftercare. By prioritizing these elements, participants can create a fulfilling and pleasurable environment that enhances both the physical and emotional aspects of their encounters. Remember, intimacy is not just about the act itself; it's about the connections forged and the memories created together.

Physical Preparation for Group Sexual Encounters

Consistent Sexual Health Practices and Testing

In the realm of group sexual encounters, the importance of consistent sexual health practices cannot be overstated. Engaging in sexual activities with multiple partners increases the risk of sexually transmitted infections (STIs) and other health concerns. Therefore, establishing a solid foundation of sexual health practices is crucial for ensuring not only personal well-being but also the safety and comfort of all participants involved.

Understanding Sexual Health

Sexual health is a multifaceted concept encompassing physical, emotional, mental, and social well-being in relation to sexuality. According to the World Health Organization (WHO), sexual health is defined as a state of physical, emotional, mental, and social well-being in relation to sexuality; it is not merely the absence of disease, dysfunction, or infirmity. This holistic view emphasizes the importance of understanding one's body, maintaining healthy relationships, and communicating effectively about sexual health.

Regular STI Testing

One of the cornerstones of consistent sexual health practices is regular STI testing. It is essential for sexually active individuals, especially those engaging in group sex, to undergo testing for STIs at regular intervals. The Centers for Disease Control and Prevention (CDC) recommend that sexually active individuals get tested at least once a year, or more frequently if they have multiple partners or engage in high-risk behaviors.

$$\text{Testing Frequency} = \begin{cases} 1 \& \text{for low-risk individuals} \\ \text{every 3-6 months} \& \text{for high-risk individuals} \end{cases} \tag{11}$$

This equation illustrates that the frequency of testing should be tailored to individual risk factors. High-risk individuals, including those with multiple partners or inconsistent condom use, should prioritize more frequent testing.

Communicating Test Results

Open communication about sexual health and testing results is vital in group sexual encounters. Before engaging in sexual activities, participants should discuss their testing history and share their results. This transparency fosters trust and ensures that everyone involved is aware of their sexual health status.

"Honesty about sexual health is not just a courtesy; it's a necessity."

When discussing test results, it's important to cover the following points:

+ The date of the last test

+ The types of STIs tested

+ Any previous infections and their treatment

+ Current sexual health practices

Utilizing Protection

Using protection, such as condoms and dental dams, is another essential practice for maintaining sexual health in group encounters. Condoms are highly effective in reducing the transmission of STIs, including HIV, gonorrhea, and chlamydia. The correct usage of condoms can be summarized in the following steps:

1. Check the expiration date and integrity of the condom package.

2. Open the package carefully to avoid tearing the condom.

3. Pinch the tip of the condom to leave space for semen.

4. Roll the condom down the length of the erect penis.

5. After ejaculation, hold the base of the condom while withdrawing to prevent spillage.

6. Dispose of the condom properly.

Addressing Common Barriers to Testing

Despite the importance of regular testing and consistent health practices, many individuals face barriers that prevent them from seeking necessary care. Common barriers include:

+ **Stigma:** Fear of judgment or discrimination can deter individuals from getting tested.

+ **Access:** Limited access to healthcare facilities or testing services can be a significant obstacle.

+ **Lack of Knowledge:** Some individuals may not be aware of the importance of regular testing or how to access services.

To combat these barriers, it is essential to create a supportive environment where individuals feel safe discussing their sexual health. This can be achieved through education, community outreach, and the promotion of accessible testing services.

Conclusion

Consistent sexual health practices and testing are fundamental components of engaging in safe and pleasurable group sexual encounters. By prioritizing regular STI testing, open communication about sexual health, and the use of protection, individuals can significantly reduce their risk of STIs and enhance their overall sexual experience. Remember, a healthy sexual life is not just about pleasure; it's about empowerment, safety, and mutual respect among all participants. By taking responsibility for your sexual health, you contribute to a more enjoyable and fulfilling group experience for everyone involved.

Safe Sex Practices in Group Settings: Protection and Consent

In the realm of group sexual encounters, the importance of safe sex practices cannot be overstated. Engaging in sexual activities with multiple partners introduces unique challenges and considerations regarding health, consent, and emotional well-being. This section will explore the fundamental aspects of safe sex practices in group settings, emphasizing the need for protection, clear communication, and mutual respect.

Understanding Protection in Group Scenarios

Protection is a cornerstone of safe sex practices, particularly in group settings where the number of sexual partners increases the potential for sexually transmitted infections (STIs). The following protective measures are essential:

+ **Condoms:** The use of condoms is one of the most effective ways to reduce the risk of STIs and unintended pregnancies. It is crucial to ensure that condoms are used consistently and correctly throughout the entire sexual encounter.

+ **Dental Dams:** For oral sex, dental dams can provide a barrier that helps prevent the transmission of infections. They are particularly important when engaging in oral-vaginal or oral-anal contact.

+ **Gloves:** When engaging in manual stimulation, using latex or nitrile gloves can help protect against the exchange of bodily fluids.

+ **Regular STI Testing:** All participants should engage in regular STI testing and share their results with each other. This transparency helps to build trust and ensures that everyone is aware of their sexual health status.

Consent: The Foundation of Group Play

Consent is the backbone of any sexual encounter, and it becomes even more critical in group scenarios. Understanding the nuances of consent in a group setting involves several key components:

+ **Enthusiastic Consent:** All participants should provide enthusiastic consent, meaning that they agree to engage in the sexual activities without any pressure or coercion. Consent should be clear, informed, and ongoing.

+ **Negotiation of Boundaries:** Before engaging in any sexual activities, it is essential to have open discussions about boundaries, desires, and limits. Each participant should feel empowered to express their preferences and establish what is acceptable and what is not.

+ **Safe Words:** Establishing safe words or signals can provide a way for participants to communicate their comfort levels during the encounter. If someone feels uncomfortable or wishes to stop, they should be able to use the safe word without hesitation.

+ **Ongoing Communication:** Consent is not a one-time agreement; it requires ongoing communication. Participants should feel free to check in with each other throughout the encounter to ensure that everyone is comfortable and enjoying the experience.

Addressing Common Problems in Group Settings

Despite the best intentions, challenges may arise in group sexual encounters. Here are some common issues and strategies for addressing them:

+ **Miscommunication:** Misunderstandings can occur regarding boundaries and consent. To mitigate this, establish clear communication channels before and during the encounter. Encourage participants to voice their thoughts and feelings openly.

+ **Pressure to Conform:** Some individuals may feel pressured to engage in activities they are uncomfortable with. It is vital to create an environment where everyone feels safe to say no and to respect those decisions without judgment.

+ **Jealousy and Insecurity:** Emotions such as jealousy can arise in group scenarios. Addressing these feelings through open dialogue can help participants navigate their emotions and reinforce trust among partners.

+ **Inconsistent Protection:** In the heat of the moment, protection may be overlooked. To prevent this, establish a routine for checking in on protection methods before engaging in sexual activities. Remind each other of the importance of using protection consistently.

Examples of Safe Sex Practices in Action

To illustrate the importance of safe sex practices in group settings, consider the following scenarios:

+ **Scenario 1:** A group of friends decides to engage in a sexual encounter. Before proceeding, they gather to discuss their boundaries, desires, and preferred protection methods. They agree to use condoms for penetrative sex and dental dams for oral sex. Each person shares their STI testing history, fostering a sense of trust and safety.

+ **Scenario 2:** During a group encounter, one participant feels uncomfortable with a specific activity. They use the established safe word, and the group immediately stops to check in. The participant expresses their discomfort, and the group discusses alternative activities that everyone is comfortable with, ensuring that consent remains a priority.

+ **Scenario 3:** After a group encounter, participants engage in aftercare, discussing their feelings and experiences. They reflect on what went well and what could be improved, reinforcing their emotional bonds and commitment to open communication in future encounters.

Conclusion

Safe sex practices in group settings are essential for ensuring the health and well-being of all participants. By prioritizing protection, consent, and open communication, individuals can create a pleasurable and safe environment for exploration. Remember, the key to fulfilling group sexual encounters lies not only in the physical pleasure but also in the emotional connection and mutual respect shared among participants. Embrace the journey of exploration with confidence, knowing that safety and consent are your guiding principles.

Ensuring Personal Hygiene and Body Care

In the context of group sexual encounters, personal hygiene and body care are paramount not only for individual health but also for creating a comfortable and pleasurable environment for all participants. This section discusses the importance of hygiene, practical steps to ensure cleanliness, and the psychological benefits of self-care in preparation for intimate group experiences.

The Importance of Hygiene

Maintaining good personal hygiene is crucial in any sexual context, but it becomes even more significant in group scenarios where multiple bodies interact closely. Poor hygiene can lead to discomfort, health issues, and even the transmission of sexually transmitted infections (STIs). According to the World Health Organization (WHO), the prevalence of STIs remains a global health concern, particularly in populations engaging in non-monogamous practices.

The psychological aspect of hygiene cannot be overlooked. Feeling clean and well-groomed enhances self-esteem and confidence, which are vital for enjoying intimate encounters. Participants who prioritize hygiene are often perceived as more attractive, fostering a more positive atmosphere.

Practical Steps for Personal Hygiene

To ensure personal hygiene and body care in group sexual encounters, consider the following practical steps:

- **Shower Beforehand:** Taking a shower before engaging in group play is one of the simplest yet most effective ways to ensure cleanliness. Use a gentle, unscented soap to avoid irritation and allergic reactions.

- **Oral Hygiene:** Fresh breath is essential in intimate settings. Brush your teeth and consider using mouthwash or breath mints. Avoid strong-smelling foods before the encounter to maintain fresh breath.

- **Grooming:** Personal grooming varies widely among individuals, but trimming or shaving pubic hair can enhance comfort and hygiene. If you choose to groom, do so carefully to avoid irritation or cuts.

- **Wear Clean, Comfortable Clothing:** Choose clothing that is clean and allows your body to breathe. Consider wearing breathable fabrics like cotton, which can help prevent moisture buildup.

- **Use Protection:** Incorporating barriers such as condoms and dental dams not only protects against STIs but also contributes to a feeling of cleanliness and safety during group encounters.

- **Hydration and Nutrition:** Staying hydrated and consuming a balanced diet can positively impact body odor and overall energy levels. Foods rich in antioxidants and probiotics can contribute to better skin and body health.

- **Post-Encounter Hygiene:** After the encounter, it is essential to clean up. Showering again can help remove bodily fluids and potential irritants, and it can also serve as a moment of self-care to reflect on the experience.

Psychological Benefits of Body Care

Engaging in body care routines can significantly enhance emotional well-being. According to research published in the *Journal of Sex Research*, individuals who engage in self-care practices report higher levels of sexual satisfaction and emotional intimacy.

$$S = f(H, C, E) \tag{12}$$

Where:

- S = Sexual satisfaction

- H = Hygiene practices

- C = Comfort level

- E = Emotional connection

This equation suggests that sexual satisfaction is a function of hygiene practices, comfort, and emotional connection, highlighting the interdependence of these factors in group sexual encounters.

Conclusion

Ensuring personal hygiene and body care is not merely a matter of cleanliness; it is a holistic approach that encompasses physical health, emotional well-being, and the creation of a positive group dynamic. By prioritizing these aspects, participants can enhance their own experiences and contribute to a more enjoyable and fulfilling environment for everyone involved. Remember, a little preparation goes a long way in maximizing pleasure and connection in group sexual encounters.

Maintaining Physical Fitness and Sexual Stamina

In the realm of group sexual encounters, maintaining physical fitness and sexual stamina is essential not only for personal enjoyment but also for the overall experience of all participants. Physical fitness can enhance sexual performance, improve endurance, and increase the ability to engage in prolonged activities. This section will discuss the importance of fitness, the challenges faced, and practical strategies to enhance stamina and overall sexual health.

The Importance of Physical Fitness

Physical fitness encompasses various components, including cardiovascular health, muscular strength, flexibility, and endurance. Each of these elements contributes to sexual performance in distinct ways:

+ **Cardiovascular Health:** Engaging in regular aerobic exercise, such as running, cycling, or swimming, improves blood circulation, which is crucial for sexual arousal and function. Enhanced blood flow can lead to improved erectile function in men and increased sensitivity in women.

+ **Muscular Strength:** Strength training not only builds muscle but also enhances endurance. Stronger muscles can lead to better control during sexual activities, allowing individuals to maintain positions and exert force when desired.

+ **Flexibility:** A flexible body can adapt to various sexual positions and movements, reducing the risk of injury and enhancing pleasure. Yoga and stretching exercises can significantly improve flexibility.

+ **Endurance:** Sexual encounters can sometimes be prolonged, especially in group settings. Building endurance through consistent cardiovascular and strength training can help individuals maintain energy levels throughout the experience.

Challenges to Maintaining Fitness

Despite the clear benefits, many individuals face challenges in maintaining their physical fitness and sexual stamina:

+ **Time Constraints:** Busy schedules can make it difficult to prioritize regular exercise. Finding time for physical activity is essential for maintaining fitness levels.

+ **Motivation:** Staying motivated to exercise can be challenging, especially when faced with fatigue or stress. Creating a supportive environment and setting achievable goals can help sustain motivation.

+ **Body Image Issues:** Concerns about body image can discourage individuals from engaging in physical activity or participating in sexual encounters. Building body positivity through self-acceptance practices can improve confidence and encourage participation.

+ **Health Conditions:** Chronic health issues or injuries can limit physical activity. Consulting with healthcare professionals to develop safe exercise plans is crucial for those facing such challenges.

Practical Strategies for Enhancing Stamina

To effectively enhance physical fitness and sexual stamina, consider the following strategies:

- **Establish a Routine:** Create a consistent exercise schedule that includes a mix of cardiovascular, strength, and flexibility training. Aim for at least 150 minutes of moderate aerobic activity each week, coupled with two days of strength training.

- **Incorporate Functional Exercises:** Focus on exercises that mimic the movements involved in sexual activity. Squats, lunges, and core exercises can improve strength and endurance in relevant muscle groups.

- **Practice Breathing Techniques:** Deep breathing exercises can enhance relaxation and stamina during sexual encounters. Techniques such as diaphragmatic breathing can help manage anxiety and improve oxygen flow to the muscles.

- **Engage in Kegel Exercises:** For individuals with vulvas, Kegel exercises strengthen the pelvic floor muscles, enhancing control and potentially leading to more intense orgasms. For individuals with penises, these exercises can help with endurance and delay ejaculation.

- **Stay Hydrated and Nourished:** Proper hydration and nutrition play a vital role in physical performance. Consuming a balanced diet rich in whole foods, lean proteins, and healthy fats can support energy levels and stamina.

- **Prioritize Rest and Recovery:** Ensure adequate sleep and recovery time between workouts. Overtraining can lead to fatigue and decreased performance, both in and out of the bedroom.

- **Explore Partner Workouts:** Engaging in physical activity with a partner can enhance connection and motivation. Consider activities such as dancing, hiking, or partner yoga to foster intimacy while improving fitness.

Example Exercises for Sexual Stamina

Here are some specific exercises that can enhance sexual stamina and overall fitness:

- **Cardiovascular Exercise:** Aim for activities like running or cycling for at least 30 minutes, 3-5 times a week. High-Intensity Interval Training (HIIT) can also be effective for building endurance in shorter time frames.

+ **Strength Training:** Incorporate compound movements such as squats, deadlifts, and bench presses into your routine. Aim for 2-3 sets of 8-12 repetitions for each exercise.

+ **Flexibility Training:** Include yoga or dynamic stretching routines at least twice a week. Focus on poses that open the hips and enhance flexibility, such as the pigeon pose and downward dog.

+ **Kegel Exercises:** For vulva owners, practice Kegels by squeezing the pelvic floor muscles as if trying to stop urination. Hold for 5 seconds, then relax. Repeat for 10-15 repetitions, 3 times a day. For penis owners, similar exercises can help strengthen pelvic muscles and control ejaculation.

Conclusion

Maintaining physical fitness and sexual stamina is a vital aspect of enjoying and maximizing pleasure in group sexual encounters. By understanding the importance of fitness, acknowledging potential challenges, and implementing practical strategies, individuals can enhance their sexual experiences. Remember that fitness is not just about performance; it is also about feeling good in your body, fostering confidence, and embracing the joy of connection with others. Empower yourself through fitness, and let your stamina carry you to new heights of pleasure.

Exploring Sensory Play and Sensual Enhancements

Sensory play involves engaging and heightening the senses to amplify pleasure and intimacy during sexual encounters. In group scenarios, sensory play can create a rich tapestry of experiences that deepen connection and enhance arousal. This section will explore the theoretical underpinnings of sensory play, common challenges, and practical examples to inspire your group encounters.

Theoretical Foundations of Sensory Play

The human body is a complex system of sensory receptors that respond to various stimuli, including touch, taste, sight, sound, and smell. Sensory play taps into these receptors, creating a multi-dimensional experience that can lead to heightened arousal and pleasure.

$$E = \sum_{i=1}^{n} S_i \tag{13}$$

Where E represents the overall experience of pleasure, and S_i denotes the individual sensory inputs (such as touch, taste, etc.). The more sensory inputs are engaged, the greater the potential for pleasure.

Theories of sexual arousal, such as the *Dual Control Model*, suggest that both excitatory and inhibitory processes govern sexual response. By focusing on sensory stimulation, participants can enhance excitatory processes, leading to increased arousal and the potential for multiple orgasms.

Common Challenges in Sensory Play

While sensory play can be incredibly rewarding, it also presents challenges:

- **Sensitivity Levels:** Individuals have varying sensitivity levels. What feels pleasurable to one person might be overwhelming or uncomfortable for another.

- **Communication:** Clear communication is essential to ensure that everyone's boundaries and preferences are respected.

- **Distraction:** In a group setting, external distractions can detract from the sensory experience. Creating a controlled environment is crucial.

- **Consent:** Engaging in sensory play requires explicit consent, particularly when introducing elements such as blindfolds or restraints.

Examples of Sensory Enhancements

Here are practical ways to incorporate sensory play into group sexual encounters:

- **Blindfolds:** Removing sight can heighten other senses. Partners can take turns being blindfolded, allowing them to focus on touch and sound. For instance, one partner may use their hands to explore another's body while the blindfolded partner expresses their pleasure through sounds.

- **Temperature Play:** Utilizing ice cubes or warm oils can create contrasting sensations on the skin. For example, running an ice cube along the spine can elicit shivers, while warm oil can provide soothing comfort. This can be particularly thrilling in a group setting where multiple partners can explore each other's reactions.

+ **Feathers and Fabrics:** Using soft feathers or various fabrics can stimulate the skin in gentle, teasing ways. Participants can take turns using these items on each other, heightening anticipation and arousal.

+ **Sound:** Incorporating music or ambient sounds can set the mood and enhance the experience. Participants may also engage in vocalizations, using moans and whispers to communicate pleasure and encouragement.

+ **Aromatherapy:** Scents can evoke powerful emotional responses. Using essential oils or scented candles can create a calming atmosphere, while certain scents may enhance arousal. For example, jasmine and ylang-ylang are known for their aphrodisiac properties.

+ **Taste:** Incorporating food into play can be both sensual and fun. Chocolate, whipped cream, or fruit can be used to explore taste and texture. Partners can feed each other, enhancing intimacy and connection.

Creating a Sensory Experience

To effectively create a sensory experience, consider the following steps:

1. **Set the Scene:** Create a comfortable and inviting environment. Use soft lighting, comfortable surfaces, and eliminate distractions.

2. **Communicate:** Discuss boundaries and preferences with all participants. Ensure everyone is comfortable with the planned sensory activities.

3. **Experiment:** Encourage exploration and playfulness. Allow participants to discover what feels good for them and their partners.

4. **Feedback:** Maintain open lines of communication throughout the experience. Encourage participants to express what they enjoy and what they would prefer to change.

5. **Aftercare:** After the experience, engage in aftercare to process the encounter and reinforce emotional connections. Discuss what felt good and what could be improved for future encounters.

In conclusion, exploring sensory play and sensual enhancements in group sexual encounters can lead to profound pleasure and connection. By understanding the theoretical foundations, addressing challenges, and implementing practical techniques, participants can create memorable experiences that celebrate their erotic selves and deepen their relationships with one another.

Utilizing Sex Toys and Props for Added Pleasure

In the vibrant landscape of group sexual encounters, the integration of sex toys and props can amplify pleasure, enhance intimacy, and create a dynamic atmosphere of exploration. This section delves into the various ways to effectively incorporate these tools into your group experiences, ensuring that every participant can ride the wave of pleasure to new heights.

Understanding the Role of Sex Toys and Props

Sex toys and props serve multiple purposes in group sexual scenarios. They can stimulate erogenous zones, facilitate varied sexual activities, and introduce elements of novelty and excitement. The use of toys can also help individuals explore their desires in a safe environment, allowing for greater expression of sexuality and creativity.

Types of Sex Toys for Group Play

1. Vibrators   Vibrators are versatile tools that can be used on oneself or shared among partners. They come in various shapes and sizes, catering to different preferences. For instance, a couple might use a wand vibrator to stimulate multiple partners simultaneously, enhancing collective pleasure.

2. Dildos   Dildos can be utilized for penetration or as props for various sexual activities. They can serve as a visual focal point, adding to the erotic atmosphere. Consider using a variety of dildos—different sizes, textures, and materials—to cater to diverse preferences within the group.

3. BDSM Gear   Incorporating BDSM props such as cuffs, blindfolds, or floggers can introduce elements of power play and sensory deprivation. These tools can heighten arousal and create a thrilling dynamic that enhances the overall experience.

4. Cock Rings and Clitoral Stimulators   These toys can enhance pleasure for both male and female participants. Cock rings can prolong erections and intensify orgasms, while clitoral stimulators can provide targeted pleasure, making them ideal for group scenarios where multiple forms of stimulation are desired.

5. Sensory Toys   Toys designed for sensory play, such as feathers, ice cubes, or temperature play props, can add an exciting layer of stimulation. These tools can be used to tease and tantalize, building anticipation and arousal among participants.

Incorporating Toys into Group Dynamics

1. Establishing Guidelines   Before introducing toys into the group setting, it is crucial to establish guidelines regarding their use. Discuss preferences, boundaries, and hygiene practices to ensure that everyone feels comfortable and safe. This conversation should include consent protocols for sharing toys and props.

2. Creating a Toy-Friendly Environment   Set up a designated area for toy storage and use. This space should be easily accessible and equipped with cleaning supplies to maintain hygiene. Creating a toy-friendly environment encourages exploration and reduces any potential stigma associated with using sex toys.

3. Encouraging Exploration   Encourage participants to explore the toys available to them. This exploration can be guided by a facilitator or can occur organically as partners engage with one another. Allowing individuals to take the lead in their pleasure can foster a sense of empowerment and confidence.

Potential Challenges and Solutions

1. Hygiene Concerns   One of the primary concerns when utilizing sex toys in group settings is hygiene. To mitigate this, ensure that all toys are cleaned before and after use. Provide access to cleaning supplies such as antibacterial wipes or toy cleaners. Discuss hygiene practices openly with all participants to foster a culture of care and respect.

2. Unequal Access to Toys   In some group dynamics, certain individuals may monopolize toys, leading to feelings of exclusion among others. To address this, establish a rotation system or encourage group sharing to ensure that everyone has the opportunity to engage with the toys.

3.   Communication Barriers   Effective communication is essential when incorporating toys into group play. Encourage participants to express their desires and boundaries regarding toy use. Utilizing a safe word or signal can help manage any discomfort that may arise during play.

Examples of Group Play Scenarios with Toys

1. The Vibrator Circle   In this scenario, participants form a circle, each equipped with a vibrator. As they explore their own bodies, they can also share their toys with one another, creating a shared experience of pleasure and connection.

2. Role-Playing with Props   Utilizing BDSM gear, participants can engage in role-playing scenarios that incorporate power dynamics. For example, one partner may take on a dominant role while using a flogger, while the others submit to the experience, enhancing the emotional and physical connection.

3. Sensory Play Stations   Set up different stations featuring various sensory toys and props. Participants can rotate through each station, exploring different sensations and experiences. This approach encourages exploration and allows individuals to discover what brings them pleasure.

Conclusion

Incorporating sex toys and props into group sexual encounters can significantly enhance pleasure and intimacy. By understanding the role of these tools, establishing clear guidelines, and fostering open communication, participants can create a rich tapestry of shared experiences. Embrace the boldness of exploration, and allow yourself and your partners to ride the wave of pleasure together, transforming group play into an unforgettable journey of connection and ecstasy.

Incorporating Erotic Massage and Sensual Touch Techniques

Erotic massage and sensual touch techniques can significantly enhance the experience of intimacy and pleasure in group sexual encounters. By creating a shared atmosphere of relaxation and connection, these practices can help participants feel more comfortable and attuned to one another's bodies, ultimately leading to heightened arousal and multiple orgasms.

Theoretical Framework

The foundation of erotic massage lies in the principles of touch, connection, and energy exchange. Touch is a powerful form of communication and can convey emotions that words often cannot. According to the work of Dr. Tiffany Field, a pioneer in the field of touch research, touch can reduce stress, increase feelings of safety, and enhance emotional bonding.

In the context of group sexual encounters, erotic massage can serve as a precursor to more explicit sexual activities. It can help participants build arousal gradually, allowing them to connect with their own bodies and those of their partners. The key is to focus on the pleasure of touch rather than the end goal of orgasm, creating a more fluid and enjoyable experience.

Common Problems in Group Settings

While incorporating erotic massage can be rewarding, certain challenges may arise:

- **Consent Issues:** It is crucial to establish clear consent before engaging in any form of touch. Participants should feel empowered to communicate their boundaries and preferences.

- **Discomfort with Intimacy:** Some individuals may feel uncomfortable with physical touch in a group setting. It's essential to create a supportive environment where everyone feels safe to express their comfort levels.

- **Unequal Attention:** In group scenarios, one partner may feel left out or overlooked during massage sessions. It's important to ensure that everyone receives equal attention and care.

- **Performance Anxiety:** Participants may worry about their skills or the reactions of others, which can hinder the experience. Emphasizing relaxation and exploration can help alleviate this anxiety.

Techniques for Erotic Massage

Here are several techniques that can be employed to create a sensual atmosphere during group encounters:

1. Setting the Scene Creating a comfortable environment is crucial for erotic massage. Dim lighting, soft music, and the use of scented oils can enhance the sensory experience. Consider using candles or essential oils like lavender or ylang-ylang to promote relaxation.

2. Communication and Consent Before beginning, gather the group to discuss preferences and boundaries. Establish a safe word or signal that anyone can use if they feel uncomfortable at any point. Encourage participants to express what feels good and what doesn't.

3. Warm-Up Techniques Start with gentle strokes to establish a connection. Use the palms of your hands to caress the back, arms, and legs of your partner, paying attention to their responses. Slow, deliberate movements help build anticipation.

4. Focus on Erogenous Zones Incorporate touch on erogenous zones, such as the neck, inner thighs, and lower back. Use varying pressure and techniques, such as kneading and circular motions, to stimulate these areas.

5. Group Dynamics Encourage participants to take turns giving and receiving massages. This can foster a sense of intimacy and connection among group members. Consider forming a circle where everyone can easily reach one another.

6. Incorporating Breathwork Encourage participants to synchronize their breathing. Deep, intentional breaths can enhance relaxation and create a shared energy flow. As tension releases, the group can collectively experience heightened arousal.

7. Using Tools and Props Introduce items such as feather ticklers, soft brushes, or massage stones to add variety to the experience. These tools can stimulate different sensations and keep the massage engaging.

8. Transitioning to Sexual Touch As the massage progresses, participants can gradually transition to more intimate touch. Encourage exploration of each other's bodies, allowing for a natural flow from massage to sexual activity.

Examples of Sensual Touch Techniques

+ **The Butterfly Stroke:** Lightly run your fingertips along the arms and shoulders of your partner, mimicking the delicate touch of a butterfly. This technique can evoke a sense of tenderness and intimacy.

+ **The Kneading Technique:** Use your palms to knead the muscles of your partner's back, applying pressure in a rhythmic motion. This technique can help release tension and promote relaxation.

+ **The Squeeze:** Gently squeeze the thighs or buttocks of your partner, alternating between firm and soft pressure. This technique can enhance arousal and create anticipation for further touch.

+ **The Circular Motion:** Use your fingertips to create small circles on the skin, particularly around sensitive areas such as the inner thighs or lower abdomen. This technique can heighten sensitivity and pleasure.

Conclusion

Incorporating erotic massage and sensual touch techniques into group sexual encounters can transform the experience, fostering deeper connections and enhancing pleasure. By prioritizing consent, communication, and a supportive environment, participants can explore their desires and boundaries in a safe and fulfilling way. As you embark on your journey of pleasure, remember that the goal is not merely to achieve orgasm, but to embrace the beauty of connection and shared intimacy.

Exploring Different Sexual Positions and Configurations in Groups

In the realm of group sexual encounters, the exploration of various sexual positions and configurations can significantly enhance pleasure and connection among participants. This section delves into the dynamics of positioning, considering both physical and emotional aspects to optimize the experience for everyone involved.

Understanding the Importance of Positioning

The choice of sexual positions in group scenarios is not merely about physical pleasure; it encompasses a range of factors including comfort, accessibility, and emotional connection. Different configurations can foster intimacy, increase arousal, and allow for greater exploration of desires.

+ **Physical Comfort:** Each participant's physical comfort is paramount. Positions that allow everyone to feel supported and relaxed can lead to a more enjoyable experience.

+ **Accessibility:** Consideration of the physical abilities of all participants is essential. Some may have mobility issues or may not be comfortable with certain positions.

+ **Emotional Connection:** Positions that allow for eye contact, touching, and closeness can enhance emotional bonds and foster a sense of safety and trust.

Common Group Configurations

1. **The Circle**: One of the simplest and most inclusive configurations is the circle. Participants sit or lie in a circle, allowing for easy access to one another. This setup encourages communication and can facilitate a variety of activities, from mutual masturbation to oral sex.

2. **The Triangle**: In a triangular configuration, three participants position themselves to create a dynamic interplay. This can be particularly stimulating as it allows for simultaneous stimulation among all parties, enhancing the sense of connection.

3. **The Sandwich**: This position involves one participant being sandwiched between two others. This configuration can create a feeling of being surrounded by pleasure, enhancing arousal through simultaneous stimulation from both sides.

4. **The Pile**: In this more chaotic arrangement, participants can intertwine in a heap, allowing for spontaneous exploration of bodies. This position encourages a playful atmosphere and can lead to unexpected pleasures.

5. **The Star**: One participant lies in the center while others surround them, engaging in various activities. This position allows for a focus on one person while still involving multiple partners, creating a sense of being adored and attended to.

Techniques for Enhancing Pleasure in Group Positions

To maximize pleasure in group scenarios, consider incorporating the following techniques:

- **Communication**: Before engaging in any position, communicate preferences and boundaries. Discuss which positions everyone is comfortable with and any specific desires. This not only ensures consent but also enhances the experience by aligning everyone's expectations.

- **Variation**: Experiment with different positions throughout the encounter. Changing configurations can maintain excitement and prevent monotony, allowing for new sensations and interactions.

- **Incorporation of Props**: Utilizing props such as cushions or sex furniture can enhance comfort and accessibility. They can also facilitate positions that might otherwise be challenging.

- **Sensory Exploration**: Encourage participants to explore each other's bodies in various positions. This can include kissing, touching, and using sex toys, which can heighten pleasure and intimacy.

Addressing Potential Challenges

While exploring different positions, it's essential to be aware of potential challenges that may arise:

- **Physical Limitations**: Be sensitive to the physical capabilities of each participant. Some may have limitations that make certain positions uncomfortable or impossible. Always prioritize comfort and safety.

- **Jealousy and Insecurity**: In group settings, feelings of jealousy or insecurity can surface. Open communication about feelings and desires can help mitigate these emotions. Establishing a culture of support and reassurance is vital.

- **Coordination**: Managing multiple bodies can sometimes lead to awkwardness. Encourage participants to move slowly and communicate openly to ensure everyone is comfortable and engaged.

Examples of Positions and Their Benefits

1. **Missionary Variation**: One partner lies on their back while others position themselves around them, either stimulating the lying partner or engaging with each other. This position promotes intimacy and allows for eye contact and connection.

2. **Doggy Style with a Twist**: In this variation, one partner kneels while another penetrates from behind, and a third partner can provide stimulation to the kneeling partner. This position allows for a mix of penetration and manual stimulation, enhancing pleasure for all involved.

3. **Cuddle Puddle**: Participants lie on their sides, facing each other or in a spooning position. This configuration allows for intimate touching and kissing, fostering emotional connection while still permitting sexual exploration.

Conclusion

Exploring different sexual positions and configurations in group encounters can significantly enhance the overall experience. By prioritizing communication, comfort, and emotional connection, participants can create a safe and pleasurable environment that allows for the exploration of desires and fantasies. Remember, the ultimate goal is to maximize pleasure and connection, so be open to experimentation and adaptability.

In the world of group sex, the possibilities are as vast as the desires of those involved. Embrace the journey, ride the waves of pleasure, and enjoy the connections that blossom in these intimate settings.

Techniques for Boosting Libido and Enhancing Arousal

In the pursuit of maximizing pleasure during group sexual encounters, understanding and enhancing libido is essential. Libido, often defined as sexual desire or drive, can fluctuate due to various factors, including stress, hormonal changes, emotional well-being, and physical health. This section explores techniques to boost libido and enhance arousal, providing practical strategies for individuals preparing for group scenarios.

Understanding Libido

Libido is influenced by a complex interplay of biological, psychological, and social factors. Theories such as the **Dual Control Model** propose that sexual arousal is governed by both excitatory and inhibitory processes. This model emphasizes the need to activate the excitatory system while minimizing inhibitory factors to enhance sexual desire.

$$\text{Sexual Arousal} = \text{Excitatory Factors} - \text{Inhibitory Factors} \qquad (14)$$

Identifying Common Barriers to Libido

Before implementing techniques to enhance libido, it is crucial to identify potential barriers:

- **Stress and Anxiety:** High levels of stress can inhibit sexual desire. Mindfulness and relaxation techniques can help mitigate these effects.

- **Hormonal Imbalances:** Fluctuations in hormones such as testosterone and estrogen can affect libido. Consulting with a healthcare provider can provide insights and potential treatments.

- **Emotional Factors:** Past traumas, relationship issues, or feelings of insecurity can dampen sexual desire. Addressing these through communication and therapy may be beneficial.

- **Physical Health:** Conditions such as diabetes, obesity, or cardiovascular issues can impact libido. A focus on overall health can improve sexual function.

Techniques for Boosting Libido

1. Mindfulness and Meditation Practicing mindfulness can enhance body awareness and reduce anxiety, leading to increased sexual desire. Techniques such as deep breathing, body scans, and focused attention can help individuals connect with their bodies, fostering a more profound sense of arousal.

2. Physical Exercise Regular physical activity is known to boost libido by increasing blood flow, enhancing body image, and releasing endorphins. Engaging in activities such as dancing, yoga, or strength training can improve overall physical health and sexual function.

3. Nutrition and Diet Certain foods are believed to enhance libido. Incorporating aphrodisiac foods such as dark chocolate, strawberries, and nuts can boost sexual desire. Additionally, maintaining a balanced diet rich in vitamins and minerals supports hormonal balance and overall health.

4. Herbal Supplements Some individuals may find that herbal supplements, such as ginseng, maca root, or tribulus terrestris, can enhance libido. However, it is essential to consult with a healthcare provider before starting any supplement regimen.

5. Sensual Exploration Encouraging sensual exploration through solo or partnered activities can increase arousal. Techniques such as erotic massage, exploring erogenous zones, and using sex toys can heighten sexual excitement and enhance overall libido.

6. Open Communication Discussing desires, fantasies, and preferences with potential partners can create a safe and stimulating environment. Open communication fosters trust and intimacy, which are critical components in enhancing libido.

7. Reducing Stress Implementing stress-reduction techniques, such as yoga, tai chi, or engaging in hobbies, can alleviate anxiety and improve sexual desire. Finding time for relaxation and self-care is vital for maintaining a healthy libido.

8. Establishing a Routine Creating a routine that includes regular intimate time with partners can help condition the body and mind for arousal. Scheduling time for intimacy, even in group settings, can signal the brain to prepare for sexual activity.

9. Limiting Alcohol and Substances While moderate alcohol consumption may lower inhibitions, excessive use can impair sexual performance and diminish libido. Being mindful of substance use is essential for maintaining sexual desire.

10. Seeking Professional Guidance If low libido persists despite efforts to enhance it, consulting with a healthcare provider or sex therapist can provide tailored strategies and support. Professional guidance can help address underlying issues and improve sexual health.

Conclusion

Boosting libido and enhancing arousal are integral components of preparing for pleasurable group sexual encounters. By understanding the factors that influence sexual desire and implementing practical techniques, individuals can cultivate a heightened sense of arousal, leading to more fulfilling experiences. Embrace the journey of exploration and connection, and remember that pleasure is a shared adventure.

Dietary Considerations for Optimal Sexual Performance

The relationship between diet and sexual performance is a topic that has garnered increasing attention in recent years. Understanding how certain foods can enhance or inhibit sexual function is crucial for anyone looking to maximize pleasure during group sexual encounters. This section will explore the dietary considerations that can lead to optimal sexual performance, focusing on the physiological and psychological effects of various nutrients and food choices.

The Role of Nutrition in Sexual Health

Nutrition plays a pivotal role in overall health, and its impact on sexual performance cannot be overstated. A well-balanced diet contributes to hormonal balance, energy levels, and blood circulation, all of which are essential for sexual arousal and performance. Nutritional deficiencies can lead to decreased libido, erectile dysfunction, and overall dissatisfaction in sexual experiences.

Key Nutrients for Sexual Performance

1. Amino Acids Amino acids, the building blocks of proteins, are crucial for the production of hormones and neurotransmitters that influence sexual desire and arousal. For instance, the amino acid *L-arginine* is known to improve blood flow by converting into nitric oxide, which relaxes blood vessels. This can enhance erectile function in men and increase sensitivity in women. Foods rich in L-arginine include:

+ Nuts (especially walnuts and almonds)

+ Seeds (pumpkin seeds and sunflower seeds)

+ Legumes (chickpeas and lentils)

+ Lean meats (turkey and chicken)

+ Seafood (shrimp and crab)

2. Vitamins and Minerals   Certain vitamins and minerals are also essential for sexual health. For example, Vitamin E is known as the "sex vitamin" because it helps maintain healthy blood circulation and hormone production. Foods high in Vitamin E include:

+ Spinach

+ Avocado

+ Nuts (especially almonds)

+ Seeds (sunflower seeds)

+ Olive oil

Zinc is another vital mineral for sexual health, particularly for men, as it plays a key role in testosterone production. Foods rich in zinc include:

+ Oysters

+ Red meat

+ Poultry

+ Beans

+ Nuts

3. Healthy Fats   Healthy fats, particularly omega-3 fatty acids, are essential for hormone production and blood flow. Incorporating sources of omega-3s into your diet can enhance sexual function. Foods rich in omega-3 fatty acids include:

+ Fatty fish (salmon, mackerel, and sardines)

+ Flaxseeds

+ Chia seeds

+ Walnuts

+ Avocado

Foods to Avoid for Optimal Performance

While certain foods can enhance sexual performance, others may hinder it. Here are some dietary choices to limit or avoid:

1. Processed Foods   High levels of sugar, unhealthy fats, and preservatives found in processed foods can lead to poor circulation, decreased libido, and overall lethargy. A diet high in processed foods can also contribute to weight gain, which may affect self-esteem and sexual confidence.

2. Alcohol   While moderate alcohol consumption can lower inhibitions and enhance sexual experiences, excessive drinking can lead to erectile dysfunction and decreased sexual arousal. It is essential to find a balance that allows for enjoyment without compromising performance.

3. High-Sodium Foods   Foods high in sodium can lead to high blood pressure, which negatively affects circulation. Poor circulation can result in diminished sexual arousal and performance. Limiting salt intake and opting for fresh, whole foods can promote better sexual health.

Hydration: The Unsung Hero

Proper hydration is often overlooked but is crucial for optimal sexual performance. Dehydration can lead to fatigue, decreased libido, and even discomfort during sexual activities. Aim to drink plenty of water throughout the day, and consider incorporating hydrating foods such as:

+ Watermelon

+ Cucumbers

+ Oranges

+ Strawberries

+ Celery

Practical Tips for Dietary Enhancement

To maximize pleasure during group sexual encounters, consider the following practical dietary tips:

1. **Plan Ahead:** Prior to group encounters, consider preparing meals that are rich in the nutrients mentioned above. A well-balanced meal can set the stage for heightened arousal and energy.

2. **Snack Smart:** If the encounter is likely to be long, opt for healthy snacks that provide sustained energy without causing fatigue. Nuts, fruits, and dark chocolate can be excellent choices.

3. **Mindful Eating:** Pay attention to how certain foods make you feel. Keep a food diary to track your dietary choices and their effects on your sexual performance.

4. **Experiment with Aphrodisiacs:** While scientific evidence may vary, many cultures believe in the power of aphrodisiac foods, such as chocolate, strawberries, and spicy peppers, to enhance sexual desire. Experimenting with these can add an element of fun and excitement to your dietary choices.

Conclusion

In conclusion, understanding the dietary considerations for optimal sexual performance is vital for anyone looking to enhance their experiences during group sexual encounters. By focusing on nutrient-rich foods that support hormonal balance and blood flow, while avoiding those that hinder performance, individuals can pave the way for more pleasurable and fulfilling sexual experiences. Remember, the journey to maximizing pleasure begins long before the encounter; it starts with what you choose to put on your plate.

Embarking on a Group Journey: Finding Partners and Creating Connections

Establishing Boundaries and Preferences

Communicating Your Boundaries and Limits to Potential Partners

In the realm of group sexual encounters, clear communication of boundaries and limits is not just a courtesy; it is a fundamental pillar that supports the entire experience. Establishing and articulating your boundaries ensures that all participants can engage in a consensual, pleasurable, and safe environment. This section explores the theory behind boundary-setting, common challenges individuals face, and practical strategies for effectively communicating your limits to potential partners.

Understanding Boundaries

Boundaries are the personal limits we establish to protect our emotional and physical well-being. They serve as guidelines for acceptable behavior and interactions, allowing individuals to navigate their desires while maintaining a sense of safety and autonomy. According to [?], boundaries are crucial in sexual relationships because they help define what is acceptable for each individual, fostering a culture of respect and consent.

Types of Boundaries

Boundaries can be categorized into several types, including:

+ **Physical Boundaries:** These pertain to personal space, touch, and physical interactions. For instance, you might specify which types of touch are acceptable or which body parts you are comfortable with others exploring.

+ **Emotional Boundaries:** These involve your feelings and emotional responses. For example, you may express a limit regarding emotional attachment or intimacy during group encounters.

+ **Time Boundaries:** These dictate how long you are willing to participate in a group encounter or how much time you need before engaging in sexual activities.

+ **Material Boundaries:** These relate to the use of personal items, such as sex toys or props, and whether you are comfortable sharing them with others.

Challenges in Communicating Boundaries

While the importance of boundaries is clear, many individuals encounter difficulties in articulating them. Some common challenges include:

+ **Fear of Rejection:** Many people worry that expressing their limits may lead to rejection or judgment from potential partners, causing them to hold back on important discussions.

+ **Social Pressure:** In group settings, the desire to fit in or please others can lead individuals to compromise their boundaries, which may result in discomfort or negative experiences.

+ **Ambiguity:** Sometimes, individuals may not fully understand their own boundaries, making it challenging to communicate them effectively. This ambiguity can stem from past experiences, cultural influences, or a lack of self-exploration.

Strategies for Effective Communication

To overcome these challenges and communicate your boundaries effectively, consider the following strategies:

1. **Self-Reflection:** Before entering a group encounter, take time to reflect on your personal boundaries. Consider what you are comfortable with and what your limits are. Journaling or discussing your thoughts with a trusted friend can help clarify your feelings.

2. **Use "I" Statements:** When expressing your boundaries, frame your statements from your perspective. For example, say "I am not comfortable with X" instead of "You can't do X." This approach reduces defensiveness and fosters open dialogue.

3. **Be Specific:** Clearly outline your boundaries to avoid misunderstandings. Instead of saying, "I don't want to go too far," specify what "too far" means to you, such as "I am comfortable with kissing but not with oral sex."

4. **Practice Active Listening:** Communication is a two-way street. Encourage your potential partners to share their boundaries as well. Validate their feelings and express appreciation for their openness. This mutual exchange builds trust and fosters a respectful environment.

5. **Establish Safe Words:** In group scenarios, having a safe word can provide an additional layer of security. A safe word allows anyone to pause or stop the activity if they feel uncomfortable, reinforcing the importance of consent and respect.

6. **Check In Regularly:** Communication should not be a one-time event. Regularly check in with your partners during the encounter to ensure everyone remains comfortable and consensual. Phrases like, "How are you feeling?" or "Is this still okay for you?" can facilitate ongoing dialogue.

Examples of Boundary Communication

To illustrate effective boundary communication, consider the following scenarios:

+ **Scenario 1: Physical Touch** - "I love being touched, but I prefer that we avoid any anal play. I'm not ready for that yet."

+ **Scenario 2: Emotional Connection** - "I enjoy group encounters, but I want to keep it casual. I'm not looking for emotional attachments right now."

+ **Scenario 3: Use of Toys** - "I'm happy to share my toys, but I'd like to discuss how we'll clean them afterward to ensure everyone's safety."

By articulating your boundaries with clarity and confidence, you empower yourself and your partners to engage in fulfilling and consensual group experiences. Remember, setting boundaries is not just about saying "no"; it is also about expressing your desires and preferences, creating a space where everyone can explore pleasure safely.

Conclusion

Communicating your boundaries and limits is an essential skill that enhances the quality of group sexual encounters. By understanding your needs, overcoming challenges, and employing effective communication strategies, you can foster a respectful and pleasurable environment for all participants. Embrace this process as a vital aspect of your sexual journey, and remember that your boundaries are a reflection of your autonomy and self-respect. In the words of [?], "Your pleasure is your own, and so are your limits."

Negotiating Boundaries and Establishing Consent in Group Scenarios

In group sexual encounters, the importance of negotiating boundaries and establishing consent cannot be overstated. These practices are foundational to ensuring that all participants feel safe, respected, and empowered to express their desires and limits. This section will delve into the theoretical underpinnings of consent, practical strategies for negotiating boundaries, and examples that illustrate the nuances of these conversations.

Theoretical Foundations of Consent

Consent is a dynamic process that requires clear communication, mutual understanding, and ongoing agreement. According to the *Affirmative Consent Model*, consent must be given freely and enthusiastically, and it can be revoked at any time. This model emphasizes that consent is not merely the absence of a "no," but rather the presence of an enthusiastic "yes." In group scenarios, where multiple individuals are involved, the complexity of consent increases, necessitating a structured approach to ensure everyone's voice is heard.

Challenges in Negotiating Boundaries

1. **Complex Dynamics**: Group settings often introduce power dynamics that can complicate consent. For example, if one partner is more dominant, others may feel pressured to agree to activities they are uncomfortable with.

2. **Miscommunication**: In the heat of the moment, communication can break down. Participants may assume that non-verbal cues are sufficient, leading to misunderstandings about boundaries and consent.

3. **Fear of Rejection**: Individuals may hesitate to express their limits due to fear of being judged or rejected by others in the group. This can lead to a lack of honest communication and potential violations of consent.

4. **Differing Expectations**: Each participant may come into the encounter with different expectations about what will happen. Without clear communication, these differing expectations can lead to discomfort or conflict.

Strategies for Effective Boundary Negotiation

To navigate these challenges, it is essential to establish a framework for negotiating boundaries and ensuring consent:

+ **Pre-Encounter Discussions**: Before engaging in group play, have open conversations about desires, limits, and expectations. This can include discussing what activities are on the table, as well as any hard or soft limits. For instance, one participant may express a hard limit against certain sexual acts, while another may have a soft limit that can be negotiated.

+ **Establishing Safe Words**: Agreeing on safe words or signals can provide a clear and immediate way for participants to communicate discomfort or the need to pause. For example, using "red" to stop and "yellow" to slow down can facilitate ongoing consent during the encounter.

+ **Check-Ins During Play**: Regularly check in with each other during the encounter to ensure that everyone is still comfortable and enjoying themselves. Simple questions like "How are you feeling?" or "Is this still good for you?" can foster a supportive atmosphere.

+ **Post-Encounter Debriefs**: After the encounter, take time to discuss what went well and any areas for improvement. This can help reinforce trust and enhance future experiences. Participants can share their feelings, any boundaries that were tested, and how they felt about the overall experience.

Examples of Boundary Negotiation

1. **Scenario A: The Enthusiastic Agreement**: In a group of four, each participant takes a moment to express their desires and limits. One person states, "I'm interested in trying oral sex, but I'm not comfortable with penetration." Another participant responds, "I'm okay with oral but would prefer to avoid any BDSM elements." This open dialogue sets a clear foundation for consent and helps everyone feel included in the decision-making process.

2. **Scenario B: The Importance of Safe Words**: During a group encounter, one participant feels overwhelmed as the activities escalate. They use the pre-agreed safe word "yellow" to indicate they need a moment to breathe. The group respects this boundary, pausing to check in and allowing the individual to regain composure before continuing.

3. **Scenario C: The Post-Encounter Reflection**: After a night of group play, participants gather to discuss their experiences. One person shares that they felt uncomfortable when a specific activity was initiated without checking in first. The group acknowledges this feedback and agrees to incorporate more check-ins in future encounters to ensure everyone feels safe and respected.

Conclusion

Negotiating boundaries and establishing consent in group sexual encounters is a vital aspect of creating a safe and pleasurable environment. By understanding the theoretical foundations of consent, acknowledging the challenges that arise in group dynamics, and employing effective strategies for communication, participants can enhance their experiences and foster deeper connections. Remember, consent is not a one-time checkbox but an ongoing dialogue that empowers everyone involved to explore their desires safely and joyfully. Embrace the conversation, honor your boundaries, and ride the wave of pleasure together.

Discussing Fantasies and Desires with Potential Partners

In the realm of group sexual encounters, open and honest communication about fantasies and desires is paramount. This dialogue not only fosters intimacy but also ensures that all participants are aligned in their expectations and comfort levels. Engaging in these discussions can be both exhilarating and daunting, yet it is a crucial step in establishing a safe and pleasurable environment.

The Importance of Communication

Communication serves as the backbone of any healthy sexual relationship, particularly in group settings where dynamics can be complex. According to the *Interpersonal Process Model of Intimacy* (Reis & Shaver, 1988), intimacy develops through self-disclosure and the partner's response. This model suggests that sharing fantasies can enhance emotional closeness and trust, making it easier to navigate the intricacies of group play.

Creating a Safe Space for Dialogue

Before diving into the specifics of desires and fantasies, it's essential to create a safe space for discussion. Here are some strategies to foster an open environment:

- **Choose the Right Setting:** Find a comfortable, private space where all participants feel at ease and can speak freely without interruptions.

- **Set Ground Rules:** Establish guidelines for the conversation, such as respecting each other's boundaries and ensuring confidentiality.

- **Encourage Active Listening:** Remind participants to listen without judgment, allowing everyone to express themselves fully.

Navigating Fantasies and Desires

When discussing fantasies, it can be helpful to structure the conversation around specific themes or scenarios. Here are some prompts to guide the dialogue:

1. **Identify Core Desires:** Ask each participant to share what they hope to experience in a group setting. This could include emotional connections, physical pleasure, or exploration of new dynamics.

2. **Explore Specific Fantasies:** Encourage participants to articulate any specific fantasies they wish to explore. For example, one might express a desire for exhibitionism, while another might fantasize about being a voyeur.

3. **Discuss Boundaries:** As fantasies are shared, it's crucial to discuss what is off-limits. This ensures that everyone feels respected and safe.

Addressing Potential Problems

While discussing fantasies can be empowering, it can also surface challenges. Here are some common issues and strategies to address them:

- **Fear of Judgment:** Participants may worry about being judged for their fantasies. Reassure everyone that all desires are valid and that the goal is to create a non-judgmental space.

- **Differing Interests:** It's possible that not everyone will share the same fantasies. Encourage compromise and collaboration, finding ways to incorporate diverse desires into the experience.

+ **Jealousy and Insecurity:** Discussing fantasies can sometimes trigger feelings of jealousy or insecurity. Acknowledge these feelings and encourage open dialogue about them, reinforcing the importance of emotional safety.

Examples of Discussion Starters

To facilitate these conversations, consider using the following examples as discussion starters:

"What is one fantasy you've always wanted to explore in a group setting?"

"How do you feel about incorporating role-play into our group experience?"

"Are there any specific boundaries you want to establish before we explore our fantasies?"

The Role of Consent in Fantasies

Consent is a crucial element when discussing and exploring fantasies. According to the *Consent Model* (Friedman et al., 2015), consent must be:

+ **Informed:** All participants should have a clear understanding of what is being proposed.

+ **Freely Given:** Consent should be given without coercion or pressure.

+ **Revocable:** Participants should feel empowered to withdraw consent at any time.

Establishing these principles ensures that the exploration of fantasies is both exciting and respectful.

Conclusion

Discussing fantasies and desires with potential partners is an essential step in preparing for group sexual encounters. By fostering open communication, creating a safe environment, and addressing potential challenges, participants can enhance their experience and deepen their connections. Embrace the excitement of sharing your fantasies, and remember that the journey toward mutual pleasure begins with understanding and respect.

Exploring Non-Monogamy and Ethical Non-Monogamy Models

Non-monogamy, a relationship style that encompasses multiple romantic or sexual relationships, challenges the traditional notion of monogamy as the only viable option for intimate partnerships. Within the realm of non-monogamy, ethical non-monogamy (ENM) has emerged as a framework that emphasizes consent, communication, and mutual respect among all parties involved. This section will explore various models of ENM, address common challenges, and provide examples to illustrate the diversity of experiences within non-monogamous relationships.

Understanding Ethical Non-Monogamy

Ethical non-monogamy refers to consensual arrangements in which individuals engage in multiple romantic or sexual relationships, with the knowledge and consent of everyone involved. Unlike cheating, which violates trust and consent, ENM is built on transparency and open communication. Key principles of ENM include:

- **Consent:** All parties must agree to the arrangement, ensuring that everyone is informed and willing to participate.

- **Communication:** Open, honest dialogue is essential for navigating emotions, desires, and boundaries.

- **Respect:** Each individual's feelings, needs, and autonomy must be honored.

Models of Ethical Non-Monogamy

There are several models of ENM, each with its unique dynamics and structures. Some of the most common models include:

- **Polyamory:** This model involves engaging in multiple romantic relationships simultaneously, where love and emotional connections are shared among partners. Polyamorous individuals often prioritize building deep emotional bonds and may practice hierarchical or non-hierarchical structures.

- **Swinging:** Swinging typically involves couples exchanging partners for sexual encounters, often in social settings or parties. The focus is primarily on sexual pleasure rather than emotional connections, and rules are often established to maintain the integrity of the primary relationship.

+ **Open Relationships:** In an open relationship, a couple maintains a primary partnership while allowing for sexual or romantic interactions with others. The boundaries and agreements regarding outside relationships can vary widely based on the couple's preferences.

+ **Relationship Anarchy:** This model rejects traditional hierarchies and labels, advocating for individualized relationships based on mutual desires and needs. Relationship anarchists prioritize autonomy and view all relationships as equally valid, regardless of their nature.

Challenges in Non-Monogamous Relationships

While ENM can be fulfilling, it is not without its challenges. Some common issues that individuals may encounter include:

+ **Jealousy:** Feelings of jealousy can arise when partners engage with others. It is crucial to address these feelings openly and constructively, as they can impact the health of all relationships involved.

+ **Time Management:** Balancing multiple relationships requires effective time management and prioritization. Partners must communicate their needs and expectations to ensure that everyone feels valued.

+ **Societal Stigma:** Non-monogamous relationships may face judgment and misunderstanding from society. This stigma can lead to feelings of isolation or pressure to conform to traditional norms.

+ **Communication Gaps:** Misunderstandings can occur if communication is not prioritized. Regular check-ins and discussions about feelings, boundaries, and desires can help mitigate this issue.

Examples of Ethical Non-Monogamy in Practice

To illustrate the diversity of ENM, consider the following examples:

+ **A Polyamorous Triad:** Three individuals, Alex, Jamie, and Taylor, form a polyamorous triad. They each share romantic and sexual relationships with one another, communicating openly about their feelings and desires. They establish boundaries regarding outside relationships and regularly check in to ensure everyone feels secure and valued.

+ **Swinging Couple:** Sam and Jordan are a couple who enjoy swinging. They attend swinger parties where they engage with other couples while maintaining their emotional bond. They set clear rules about what activities are acceptable and prioritize their communication before and after events to address any feelings that may arise.

+ **Open Relationship:** Mia and Chris have an open relationship where they maintain their primary partnership while exploring sexual connections with others. They discuss their experiences and feelings regularly, ensuring that their primary relationship remains strong and fulfilling.

+ **Relationship Anarchy:** Taylor embraces relationship anarchy, engaging in various connections without defining them by traditional labels. They prioritize communication and mutual respect, allowing relationships to evolve organically based on the desires of all involved.

Conclusion

Exploring non-monogamy and ethical non-monogamy models opens up a world of possibilities for individuals seeking to expand their sexual and emotional horizons. By prioritizing consent, communication, and respect, individuals can navigate the complexities of multiple relationships while fostering deeper connections with themselves and their partners. Whether through polyamory, swinging, open relationships, or relationship anarchy, the key to success lies in understanding one's desires, establishing clear boundaries, and engaging in open dialogue. Embracing non-monogamy can lead to enriched experiences, personal growth, and a broader understanding of love and intimacy.

Utilizing Online Platforms and Communities for Finding Group Partners

In the modern era, the internet has revolutionized the way we connect, explore, and engage in sexual encounters, particularly in group settings. The utilization of online platforms and communities presents a unique opportunity for individuals seeking to expand their sexual horizons and find partners who share similar desires. This section explores the various online avenues available, the potential challenges, and practical tips for navigating these spaces effectively.

Exploring Online Platforms

The digital landscape offers a plethora of options for those interested in group sexual encounters. From dedicated dating apps to social media groups, individuals can find like-minded partners with relative ease. Notable platforms include:

+ **Swinger Dating Sites:** Websites such as AdultFriendFinder, SwingLifestyle, and FetLife cater specifically to individuals interested in non-monogamous relationships and group encounters. These platforms allow users to create profiles, share their interests, and connect with potential partners.

+ **Social Media Groups:** Facebook and Reddit host numerous groups dedicated to alternative lifestyles, including swinging and polyamory. These communities provide a space for discussion, advice, and the opportunity to meet potential partners.

+ **Dating Apps:** Apps like Feeld and OkCupid allow users to specify their interest in group play and non-monogamous arrangements, making it easier to find compatible partners.

Theoretical Framework: Online Interaction and Sexual Exploration

The theory of *social penetration* suggests that relationships develop through a gradual process of self-disclosure and intimacy. In online platforms, individuals can curate their profiles to present their sexual preferences and boundaries, facilitating deeper connections. This theory is particularly relevant in group scenarios, where multiple individuals must navigate their desires and limits.

$$\text{Intimacy} = f(\text{Self-Disclosure}, \text{Reciprocity}) \qquad (15)$$

Where: - Intimacy represents the closeness developed between partners. - Self-Disclosure refers to the sharing of personal information and desires. - Reciprocity indicates the mutual exchange of information, fostering trust.

Challenges of Online Platforms

While online platforms provide access to potential partners, they also come with challenges that require careful navigation:

+ **Misrepresentation:** Online profiles may not always accurately reflect an individual's true self. It is crucial to engage in open communication and verify the authenticity of potential partners before meeting.

- **Safety Concerns:** The anonymity of the internet can lead to safety issues. Users should prioritize their safety by arranging initial meetings in public spaces and informing trusted friends of their whereabouts.

- **Emotional Vulnerability:** Group dynamics can intensify feelings of jealousy and insecurity. It is essential to establish clear communication and boundaries before engaging in group encounters to mitigate these feelings.

Practical Tips for Finding Group Partners Online

To maximize the potential of online platforms for finding group partners, consider the following strategies:

- **Create an Honest Profile:** Clearly articulate your desires, boundaries, and what you are looking for in a group encounter. Honesty will attract partners who align with your interests.

- **Engage Actively:** Participate in discussions, share experiences, and offer support within online communities. This engagement fosters relationships and builds trust among potential partners.

- **Establish Clear Communication:** Use direct and open communication to discuss boundaries, desires, and expectations with potential partners. Consider using *negotiation frameworks* to facilitate these discussions.

- **Attend Online Events:** Many platforms host virtual meet-and-greets or workshops focused on group dynamics. Participating in these events can help you connect with others interested in group encounters.

Examples of Successful Online Connections

Consider the following scenarios where individuals successfully utilized online platforms to find group partners:

- **Case Study 1:** Alex, a 30-year-old bisexual individual, joined a local swinger group on Facebook. After engaging in discussions and sharing their interests, Alex attended a virtual meet-up. This led to connections with several like-minded individuals, ultimately resulting in a successful group encounter.

+ **Case Study 2:** Jamie, a 28-year-old non-binary person, used the Feeld app to connect with potential partners. By being transparent about their desires for group play and establishing clear boundaries, Jamie was able to form a group that prioritized consent and communication, leading to a fulfilling experience.

In conclusion, online platforms and communities offer valuable resources for individuals seeking group sexual encounters. By understanding the dynamics of online interactions, addressing potential challenges, and employing effective strategies, individuals can navigate these spaces confidently and safely. Embrace the opportunity to explore your desires and connect with others who share your passion for pleasure.

Joining Swinger Clubs and Erotic Events for Group Encounters

Joining swinger clubs and attending erotic events can be an exhilarating way to explore group sexual encounters. These spaces offer opportunities for connection, exploration, and pleasure in a consensual and often community-oriented environment. However, navigating these venues requires understanding, preparation, and a commitment to communication and consent.

Understanding Swinger Culture

Swinger clubs and erotic events are part of a broader culture that values open relationships and sexual exploration. These communities often emphasize the importance of consent, communication, and respect. The foundational principles include:

+ **Consent:** All activities must be consensual among all parties involved. This is non-negotiable in creating a safe and enjoyable environment.

+ **Communication:** Open and honest communication about desires, boundaries, and expectations is essential. This includes discussing what participants are comfortable with and what they wish to avoid.

+ **Respect:** Respect for personal boundaries, as well as for the feelings and desires of others, is crucial to maintaining a positive atmosphere.

Finding the Right Club or Event

Not all swinger clubs or erotic events are the same. It is important to research and find a venue that aligns with your values and desires. Consider the following factors:

+ **Community Reputation:** Look for clubs or events with positive reviews and a reputation for safety and inclusivity. Online forums and social media groups can provide insights into the experiences of others.

+ **Inclusivity:** Choose venues that welcome diverse sexual orientations, identities, and relationship styles. A welcoming environment enhances the experience for everyone involved.

+ **Atmosphere:** Visit the club's website or attend an introductory event to gauge the atmosphere. Some clubs may focus on a party vibe, while others may prioritize intimacy and connection.

Preparing for Your Visit

Preparation is key to ensuring a positive experience at swinger clubs or erotic events. Here are some important considerations:

+ **Personal Hygiene:** Prioritize cleanliness and grooming before attending. This shows respect for yourself and others and enhances the overall experience.

+ **Dress Code:** Many clubs have specific dress codes that encourage sensuality and self-expression. Choose an outfit that makes you feel confident and attractive.

+ **Safety Practices:** Familiarize yourself with the club's safety protocols, including rules around condom use and sexual health. Bring your own protection to ensure your safety and that of your partners.

Navigating the Space

Once you arrive at a swinger club or erotic event, it's essential to navigate the space with confidence and awareness. Consider the following tips:

+ **Observe First:** Take time to observe the dynamics and interactions before jumping into activities. This can help you gauge the atmosphere and understand the social norms of the venue.

+ **Engage in Conversation:** Start conversations with other attendees to build rapport and establish connections. Use open-ended questions to encourage dialogue about interests and boundaries.

+ **Establish Boundaries:** Clearly communicate your boundaries to potential partners. This includes discussing what activities you are open to and what you wish to avoid.

Handling Emotions and Dynamics

Group encounters can evoke a range of emotions, from excitement to jealousy. It's important to be prepared for these feelings:

+ **Stay Grounded:** Practice mindfulness techniques to stay present and grounded during your experience. This can help you manage any overwhelming emotions that arise.

+ **Check-In with Partners:** Regularly check in with your partners during the encounter to ensure everyone is comfortable and enjoying themselves. This fosters a supportive environment.

+ **Aftercare:** After the event, engage in aftercare with your partners to process the experience and reinforce emotional connections. This can include cuddling, discussing feelings, or simply spending quiet time together.

Example Scenario

To illustrate the process, consider the following example:

You and your partner decide to attend a local swinger club after researching various options. You choose a venue known for its welcoming atmosphere and strong emphasis on consent. Before attending, you have an open discussion about your boundaries and desires, agreeing on a safe word to use if either of you feels uncomfortable.

Upon arrival, you take time to observe the interactions around you. You engage in conversation with a few other attendees, sharing your interests and gauging their comfort levels. As you explore the space, you establish connections with others, communicating your boundaries clearly.

After a fulfilling evening of exploration, you both return home and engage in aftercare, discussing what you enjoyed and any emotions that arose during the experience. This reflection not only strengthens your bond but also prepares you for future encounters.

Conclusion

Joining swinger clubs and attending erotic events can be a thrilling way to explore group sexual encounters. By understanding the culture, preparing adequately, and prioritizing communication and consent, you can create a fulfilling and pleasurable experience. Remember, every encounter is an opportunity for growth, connection, and exploration of your desires in a safe and consensual environment.

Attending BDSM and Kink Communities for Group Play

Engaging in group sexual encounters within BDSM and kink communities can be an exhilarating and deeply fulfilling experience. These communities often emphasize consent, communication, and safety, providing a supportive environment for exploring diverse sexual expressions. To navigate these spaces effectively, it's essential to understand the unique dynamics and protocols that govern BDSM and kink play.

Understanding BDSM and Kink Culture

BDSM, which stands for Bondage, Discipline, Dominance, Submission, Sadism, and Masochism, encompasses a wide range of practices that involve power exchange and consensual exploration of physical and psychological sensations. Kink refers to any unconventional sexual practices that may not fall under the BDSM umbrella but still involve elements of fantasy and role-play.

The culture surrounding BDSM and kink communities is characterized by a strong emphasis on the principles of **Safe, Sane, and Consensual (SSC)** or **Risk-Aware Consensual Kink (RACK)**. These guiding principles encourage participants to engage in practices that prioritize safety and informed consent, ensuring that all parties involved are aware of the risks and have mutually agreed to the activities.

Finding the Right Community

To participate in group play, it's crucial to find a community that aligns with your interests and values. Here are some steps to consider:

- **Research Local Groups:** Use online platforms, social media, and community boards to identify local BDSM and kink groups. Websites like FetLife can be valuable resources for connecting with others who share similar interests.

+ **Attend Workshops and Events:** Many communities host educational workshops and social events. These gatherings provide opportunities to learn about BDSM practices, meet potential partners, and establish connections in a non-sexual environment.

+ **Join a Dungeon or Club:** Many cities have dedicated BDSM dungeons or clubs that host regular events. These spaces often have established protocols for safety and consent, making them ideal for group encounters.

Establishing Consent and Boundaries

In BDSM and kink communities, consent is paramount. Before engaging in any group play, it's essential to have clear and open discussions about boundaries, desires, and limits with all participants. Here are some strategies for effective communication:

+ **Pre-Play Negotiation:** Before any activities begin, negotiate specific roles, limits, and safe words. This negotiation should include discussions about what each participant is comfortable with and any hard limits that should not be crossed.

+ **Utilizing Safe Words:** Establishing safe words is crucial in BDSM play. A common system includes using a traffic light system where *green* indicates "go," *yellow* means "slow down," and *red* signifies "stop immediately." Ensure that everyone understands and respects these signals.

+ **Check-Ins:** During play, regular check-ins can help maintain comfort levels. Simple questions like "How are you feeling?" or "Is this okay?" can foster a sense of safety and care among participants.

Navigating Group Dynamics

Group dynamics in BDSM and kink scenarios can vary significantly from one encounter to another. Understanding the roles and relationships among participants is essential for a positive experience. Here are some common dynamics to consider:

+ **Top/Bottom Dynamics:** In BDSM, roles are often defined as "top" (the person who exerts control or administers sensations) and "bottom" (the person who receives sensations). In group settings, these roles can shift and change, so clarity is key.

+ **Switching Roles:** Many individuals identify as "switches," meaning they enjoy both dominant and submissive roles. Being open to switching can enhance the experience and allow for a more fluid exploration of power dynamics.

+ **Group Hierarchies:** In some BDSM settings, established hierarchies may exist, especially in larger groups or communities. Understanding these dynamics can help navigate interactions and ensure respectful engagement.

Addressing Common Challenges

While BDSM and kink communities offer thrilling opportunities for exploration, they also present challenges that must be addressed:

+ **Jealousy and Insecurity:** In group settings, feelings of jealousy or insecurity can arise, particularly if one partner seems to receive more attention. Open communication and reaffirming emotional connections can help mitigate these feelings.

+ **Miscommunication:** Misunderstandings can lead to discomfort or even harm. Maintaining clear communication before, during, and after play is essential to ensure that everyone's needs are met and respected.

+ **Aftercare Needs:** Aftercare is a critical component of BDSM play, particularly in group scenarios where emotional and physical intensity can be high. Discuss aftercare preferences with partners beforehand, ensuring that everyone knows how to support each other post-play.

Examples of Group Play Scenarios

To illustrate the possibilities within BDSM and kink communities, consider the following examples of group play scenarios:

+ **Bondage Workshops:** Participants can engage in group bondage sessions where they practice tying each other up under the guidance of an experienced instructor. This setting fosters learning, connection, and shared pleasure.

+ **Sensory Deprivation Games:** In a group setting, participants can explore sensory deprivation through blindfolds, earplugs, or restraints, enhancing the thrill of anticipation and heightening sensations.

+ **Role-Playing Scenarios:** Groups can engage in elaborate role-playing scenarios, such as a teacher-student dynamic or a master-servant relationship, allowing for exploration of fantasies in a safe and consensual manner.

Conclusion

Attending BDSM and kink communities for group play can be a transformative experience, offering opportunities for pleasure, connection, and personal growth. By prioritizing consent, communication, and emotional safety, participants can navigate these encounters with confidence and enthusiasm. Embrace the journey, explore your desires, and remember that the key to a fulfilling experience lies in mutual respect and understanding.

Understanding and Addressing Power Dynamics in Group Scenarios

In group sexual encounters, power dynamics play a significant role in shaping the experience for all participants. Understanding these dynamics is crucial for creating a safe, consensual, and pleasurable environment. Power dynamics can manifest in various forms, influenced by factors such as gender, sexual orientation, experience level, and personal insecurities. This section explores the nature of power dynamics, the potential issues that can arise, and strategies for addressing them effectively.

The Nature of Power Dynamics

Power dynamics refer to the ways in which power is distributed and exercised within interpersonal relationships. In group sexual scenarios, these dynamics can be explicit or implicit and may shift throughout the encounter. Some common types of power dynamics include:

+ **Dominance and Submission:** These dynamics often involve one partner taking a more dominant role while others assume submissive positions. This can enhance arousal for some participants but requires clear communication and consent.

+ **Experience Levels:** Participants with varying levels of sexual experience may unintentionally create power imbalances. More experienced individuals may inadvertently dominate discussions or activities, leading to feelings of inadequacy among less experienced partners.

+ **Social and Cultural Influences:** Societal norms and cultural backgrounds can shape perceptions of power in sexual encounters. For example, traditional gender roles may influence expectations around who takes the lead in sexual situations.

+ **Emotional Vulnerability:** Participants may bring emotional baggage into group encounters, affecting their ability to assert boundaries. Those who are more emotionally vulnerable may find themselves in subordinate positions, even if this is not their intention.

Potential Problems Arising from Power Dynamics

Power imbalances can lead to several issues in group sexual encounters:

+ **Lack of Consent:** If one partner dominates the interaction, others may feel pressured to acquiesce, leading to situations where consent is not fully informed or enthusiastic.

+ **Resentment and Jealousy:** Unequal power dynamics can foster feelings of resentment or jealousy among participants, particularly if one individual receives more attention or affection.

+ **Emotional Distress:** Participants may experience emotional distress if they feel marginalized or disempowered. This can lead to negative associations with future group encounters or affect their overall sexual well-being.

+ **Miscommunication:** Power dynamics can complicate communication, making it difficult for participants to express their needs, desires, or concerns openly.

Strategies for Addressing Power Dynamics

To ensure that power dynamics enhance rather than hinder the experience, participants should consider the following strategies:

+ **Establish Clear Communication:** Before engaging in group play, participants should discuss their boundaries, preferences, and any existing power dynamics. Open communication fosters trust and helps everyone feel heard and respected.

+ **Create a Safe Word or Signal:** Establishing a safe word or signal can empower participants to communicate discomfort or the need to pause the activity. This practice reinforces the importance of consent and allows individuals to reclaim their power if they feel overwhelmed.

+ **Encourage Equal Participation:** Facilitate an environment where all participants have the opportunity to voice their desires and boundaries. This can be achieved through group discussions or check-ins during the encounter.

+ **Acknowledge and Address Imbalances:** Participants should be aware of their own privileges and biases, actively working to address any unintentional imbalances. This may involve stepping back to allow others to take the lead or encouraging quieter partners to express their needs.

+ **Foster Emotional Support:** Building emotional connections within the group can help mitigate the effects of power imbalances. Engaging in aftercare practices, such as cuddling or discussing the experience, can reinforce a sense of community and support.

Examples of Power Dynamics in Action

Consider the following scenarios to illustrate how power dynamics can manifest and be addressed:

+ **Scenario 1: The Experienced Leader**
In a group where one participant is significantly more experienced, they may unintentionally dominate the conversation about preferences and boundaries. To address this, the group can implement a round-robin discussion format, allowing each participant to share their thoughts and desires without interruption.

+ **Scenario 2: The Shy Participant**
A quieter individual may feel overshadowed by more vocal partners, leading to feelings of inadequacy. To empower this participant, the group can create a supportive atmosphere by actively inviting them to share their thoughts and reassuring them that their contributions are valued.

+ **Scenario 3: The Power Exchange**
In a BDSM context, power dynamics are often explicitly negotiated. However, it is essential to regularly check in with all participants to ensure

that everyone feels comfortable and that the power exchange remains consensual. Establishing clear safe words and aftercare practices can help maintain emotional safety.

Conclusion

Understanding and addressing power dynamics in group sexual encounters is essential for fostering a safe and pleasurable environment. By recognizing the various forms of power that can emerge, participants can work collaboratively to create a space where everyone's desires and boundaries are respected. Open communication, active participation, and emotional support are key components in navigating these dynamics, ultimately leading to more fulfilling and enjoyable group experiences.

Assessing Personal Compatibility: Emotional and Sexual Chemistry

In the realm of group sexual encounters, understanding personal compatibility is crucial for fostering a harmonious and pleasurable experience. Emotional and sexual chemistry between partners can significantly enhance the overall dynamic, making it imperative to assess these elements before engaging in group play. This section delves into the theories surrounding emotional and sexual chemistry, common problems that may arise, and practical examples to guide individuals in evaluating compatibility.

Theoretical Framework

Emotional and sexual chemistry can be understood through several psychological and biological theories. One prominent theory is the **Attachment Theory**, which posits that our early relationships with caregivers shape how we connect with others throughout life. In adult relationships, attachment styles—secure, anxious, and avoidant—can influence how individuals engage in emotional and sexual intimacy.

$$\text{Compatibility Index} = \frac{E + S}{2} \tag{16}$$

Where:

- E = Emotional compatibility score (rated from 1 to 10)

- S = Sexual compatibility score (rated from 1 to 10)

A higher Compatibility Index indicates a stronger potential for positive interactions in group settings.

Identifying Emotional Chemistry

Emotional chemistry is characterized by a deep sense of connection, mutual understanding, and shared values. To assess emotional compatibility, consider the following factors:

- **Communication Styles:** How do you and your potential partners express thoughts and feelings? Open and honest communication fosters emotional intimacy.

- **Shared Values and Beliefs:** Common values regarding relationships, sexuality, and consent can enhance emotional compatibility. Discuss these topics openly before engaging in group play.

- **Empathy and Support:** Evaluate how partners respond to each other's emotions. A supportive environment encourages vulnerability and connection.

Identifying Sexual Chemistry

Sexual chemistry, on the other hand, relates to the physical attraction and sexual compatibility between partners. Key factors to consider include:

- **Attraction Levels:** Assess mutual attraction. Attraction can be influenced by physical appearance, body language, and energy.

- **Sexual Preferences:** Discuss sexual desires, kinks, and preferences. Understanding what each partner enjoys can significantly enhance sexual chemistry.

- **Physical Compatibility:** Consider how well partners' bodies mesh during sexual activities. Different body types may require adjustments for optimal pleasure.

Common Problems in Assessing Compatibility

Despite the importance of emotional and sexual chemistry, several challenges may arise during the assessment process:

+ **Miscommunication:** Inadequate communication can lead to misunderstandings regarding desires and boundaries. It is essential to foster an environment where all partners feel safe to express themselves.

+ **Differing Expectations:** Partners may have different expectations about the nature of the relationship or group encounter. Clarifying intentions beforehand can mitigate potential conflicts.

+ **Jealousy and Insecurity:** Emotional insecurities can cloud judgment and affect compatibility assessments. Addressing these feelings openly with partners is vital for maintaining a healthy dynamic.

Practical Examples

To illustrate the assessment of emotional and sexual chemistry, consider the following scenarios:

Scenario 1: Emotional Compatibility Alice and Bob are considering engaging in a group encounter. Before proceeding, they discuss their attachment styles. Alice identifies as securely attached, while Bob admits to being more avoidant. They explore how this difference may affect their emotional connection in a group setting. They decide to establish clear communication protocols to ensure both feel comfortable expressing their needs.

Scenario 2: Sexual Compatibility Carmen, Diego, and Eve are exploring group play. They hold a candid discussion about their sexual preferences, including kinks and boundaries. Carmen expresses her interest in BDSM, while Diego prefers more traditional sexual activities. They negotiate a plan that incorporates elements of both preferences, ensuring everyone feels included and excited about the experience.

Conclusion

Assessing personal compatibility through emotional and sexual chemistry is a vital step in preparing for group sexual encounters. By understanding the theoretical frameworks, identifying key factors, addressing common problems, and utilizing practical examples, individuals can navigate the complexities of compatibility with confidence. Ultimately, fostering strong emotional and sexual connections enhances the pleasure and satisfaction of all participants, paving the way for fulfilling group experiences.

Establishing Trust and Emotional Connection in Group Dynamics

In the realm of group sexual encounters, establishing trust and emotional connection is paramount. These elements not only enhance the pleasure of the experience but also create a safe space where individuals can explore their desires without fear or hesitation. Trust is the foundation upon which all intimate relationships are built, and in group dynamics, it becomes even more crucial due to the complexities of multiple interactions and the potential for emotional vulnerabilities.

The Importance of Trust

Trust can be defined as the belief in the reliability, truth, ability, or strength of someone or something. In a group sexual context, trust involves several dimensions:

- **Reliability:** Partners must feel confident that their needs and boundaries will be respected.

- **Emotional Safety:** Participants should feel secure in expressing their desires, fears, and boundaries without judgment.

- **Consistency:** Trust is built over time through consistent behavior and communication.

The establishment of trust can be supported by various theories, including the *Social Exchange Theory*, which posits that relationships are formed based on the perceived benefits and costs. In group scenarios, individuals weigh the emotional and physical risks against the potential for pleasure and connection.

$$\text{Trust} = \frac{\text{Perceived Benefits}}{\text{Perceived Costs}} \qquad (17)$$

This equation illustrates that as perceived benefits increase, so does the likelihood of trust being established, provided that the perceived costs remain manageable.

Building Emotional Connections

Emotional connections in group dynamics can be fostered through intentional practices that promote vulnerability and authenticity. Here are several strategies to enhance emotional bonds among group members:

+ **Open Communication:** Encourage participants to share their thoughts, feelings, and boundaries openly. This can be facilitated through pre-play discussions where everyone has the opportunity to express their desires and concerns.

+ **Active Listening:** Practicing active listening fosters empathy and understanding. Encourage group members to reflect back what they hear, validating each person's feelings and perspectives.

+ **Shared Experiences:** Engaging in activities that promote bonding, such as group workshops or ice-breaking games, can enhance emotional intimacy. These shared experiences create a sense of camaraderie and trust.

+ **Aftercare Practices:** Aftercare is crucial in maintaining emotional connections post-encounter. This can involve cuddling, discussing the experience, or simply checking in with each other's emotional state. Acknowledging the shared journey helps reinforce bonds.

Addressing Challenges in Trust and Connection

Despite the best intentions, challenges may arise in establishing trust and emotional connection within group dynamics. Common issues include:

+ **Jealousy and Insecurity:** Feelings of jealousy can disrupt trust and connection. It is essential to address these feelings openly and constructively. Implementing regular check-ins can help mitigate these emotions.

+ **Miscommunication:** Misunderstandings can lead to breaches of trust. Clear and concise communication protocols, including the use of safe words and consent check-ins, can help alleviate these issues.

+ **Differing Expectations:** Each participant may have different expectations regarding the encounter. Establishing a group agreement that outlines everyone's desires and boundaries can help align expectations and foster trust.

Examples of Trust-Building Activities

To illustrate how trust and emotional connection can be nurtured in group dynamics, consider the following examples:

+ **Trust Exercises:** Simple trust-building exercises, such as trust falls or guided partner activities, can help participants become more comfortable with each other. These activities encourage vulnerability and reliance on one another.

+ **Group Discussions:** Organizing a group discussion focused on past experiences, desires, and fears can help participants connect on a deeper level. Sharing personal stories fosters empathy and understanding.

+ **Feedback Sessions:** After a group encounter, hold a feedback session where participants can share their experiences and feelings. This practice not only promotes emotional connection but also enhances future encounters by addressing any issues that arose.

Conclusion

In conclusion, establishing trust and emotional connection in group dynamics is essential for maximizing pleasure and ensuring a safe, consensual experience. By prioritizing open communication, active listening, and intentional bonding activities, participants can create a nurturing environment that allows for exploration and fulfillment. Challenges such as jealousy and miscommunication can be effectively managed through proactive strategies, reinforcing the bonds of trust that enhance the overall experience. Remember, the journey of pleasure is best traveled together, with trust as your compass and connection as your guide.

Communication and Consent in Group Scenarios

Effective Communication Strategies for Group Sexual Encounters

Effective communication is the cornerstone of enjoyable and fulfilling group sexual encounters. In a setting where multiple individuals are involved, the dynamics of communication can become complex. This section will explore practical strategies for ensuring that all participants feel heard, respected, and engaged in the experience.

1. The Importance of Clear Communication

Communication in group settings serves several critical functions:

+ **Establishing Consent:** Clear dialogue is essential for gaining and maintaining consent among all participants. This includes discussing boundaries, desires, and any limitations before engaging in sexual activities.

- **Building Trust:** Open lines of communication foster an environment of trust, where individuals feel safe expressing their needs and concerns.

- **Enhancing Pleasure:** Effective communication about preferences and desires can lead to a more pleasurable experience for everyone involved.

- **Navigating Conflict:** Disagreements or misunderstandings can arise in group scenarios. Being able to communicate effectively can help resolve issues quickly and amicably.

2. Strategies for Effective Communication

2.1 Pre-Encounter Discussions   Before the group encounter, it is vital to have open discussions about expectations. Here are some strategies to facilitate this:

- **Set a Meeting:** Arrange a time for all participants to meet (in person or virtually) before the encounter. This allows everyone to discuss their desires, boundaries, and any concerns.

- **Use "I" Statements:** Encourage participants to express their feelings using "I" statements (e.g., "I feel comfortable with..." or "I would like to explore..."). This approach reduces defensiveness and promotes understanding.

- **Discuss Boundaries:** Clearly outline personal boundaries and respect those of others. Use a boundary checklist to facilitate this process, where individuals can indicate their limits on various activities.

2.2 Consent Protocols   Establishing consent protocols is crucial in group dynamics. Consider the following:

- **Explicit Consent:** Ensure that consent is obtained explicitly from all parties involved. This can be verbal or through a written agreement outlining the activities everyone is comfortable with.

- **Safe Words:** Implement safe words that anyone can use to pause or stop the encounter if they feel uncomfortable. This can be a simple word like "red" for stop and "yellow" for slow down.

- **Continuous Consent:** Remind participants that consent is an ongoing process. Check in with each other throughout the encounter to ensure everyone is still comfortable and enjoying themselves.

2.3 Active Listening Techniques   Active listening is an essential component of effective communication. Here are some techniques to enhance this skill:

+ **Reflective Listening:** Repeat back what someone has said to ensure understanding. For example, "What I hear you saying is that you're interested in trying..." This confirms that you are engaged and valuing their input.

+ **Non-Verbal Cues:** Pay attention to body language and other non-verbal signals. Nods, eye contact, and posture can indicate comfort or discomfort, even if words are not spoken.

+ **Avoid Interrupting:** Allow each participant to express themselves fully before responding. This fosters a respectful environment where everyone feels valued.

2.4 Addressing Jealousy and Insecurity   In group scenarios, feelings of jealousy or insecurity may arise. Here's how to handle these emotions through communication:

+ **Acknowledge Feelings:** Encourage participants to voice their feelings of jealousy or insecurity without fear of judgment. Acknowledging these feelings can help normalize them and reduce their power.

+ **Discuss Solutions:** Once feelings are expressed, engage in a constructive dialogue about how to address them. For instance, if one partner feels neglected, discuss ways to ensure everyone feels included.

+ **Reassurance:** Provide reassurance to each other. Simple affirmations of love, attraction, and desire can help mitigate feelings of insecurity.

3. Examples of Effective Communication in Action

To illustrate these strategies, consider the following scenarios:

Scenario 1: Setting Boundaries   Before a group encounter, participants gather to discuss their limits. One participant states, "I'm comfortable with kissing and touching, but I'm not ready for penetration." The group acknowledges this boundary, and everyone agrees to respect it, ensuring a safe environment.

Scenario 2: Using Safe Words During a group encounter, one participant feels overwhelmed and uses the safe word "yellow." The group pauses and checks in with them, allowing for a moment of reflection and reassessment of comfort levels.

Scenario 3: Addressing Jealousy After a particularly intense encounter, one participant expresses feelings of jealousy regarding another's attention. The group engages in an open discussion about these feelings, offering support and reassurance to one another, ultimately strengthening their connections.

4. Conclusion

Effective communication in group sexual encounters is not just beneficial; it is essential. By prioritizing clear dialogue, establishing consent protocols, and actively listening to one another, participants can create an environment of trust and pleasure. Remember, the goal is to ensure that everyone feels safe, respected, and fulfilled. By implementing these strategies, you can navigate the complexities of group dynamics while maximizing the enjoyment of all involved.

Maintaining Open Lines of Communication with Group Partners

Effective communication is the cornerstone of any successful sexual encounter, especially in the complex dynamics of group scenarios. Maintaining open lines of communication with group partners is essential for fostering trust, ensuring consent, and enhancing pleasure. This section will explore the importance of communication, common challenges, and practical strategies to keep conversations flowing smoothly.

The Importance of Communication

Communication serves several vital functions in group sexual encounters:

- **Establishing Consent:** Clear communication about desires, boundaries, and consent ensures that all participants feel safe and respected. This is particularly important in group settings where individuals may have varying comfort levels and expectations.

- **Building Trust:** Open dialogue fosters an environment of trust, allowing partners to express their needs and concerns without fear of judgment. Trust is critical for enhancing intimacy and connection among participants.

- **Enhancing Pleasure:** By discussing preferences, fantasies, and feedback, partners can tailor their experiences to maximize pleasure for everyone involved. This collaborative approach can lead to more fulfilling and enjoyable encounters.

- **Addressing Issues:** Open communication allows for the timely identification and resolution of any issues or discomforts that may arise during the encounter. This proactive approach can prevent misunderstandings and negative experiences.

Common Challenges in Communication

While the importance of communication is clear, several challenges can hinder effective dialogue in group scenarios:

- **Fear of Vulnerability:** Participants may hesitate to express their desires or boundaries due to fear of vulnerability or judgment. This can lead to unspoken assumptions and unmet needs.

- **Misinterpretation:** Non-verbal cues and body language can be easily misinterpreted in the heat of the moment, leading to confusion and potential discomfort.

- **Overwhelm:** In a group setting, the presence of multiple partners can be overwhelming, making it difficult to focus on individual communication. Participants may struggle to articulate their needs amidst the excitement.

- **Power Dynamics:** Unequal power dynamics can affect communication, with some individuals feeling less empowered to voice their opinions or desires. This can create an imbalance that impacts the overall experience.

Strategies for Maintaining Open Communication

To overcome these challenges and maintain open lines of communication, consider the following strategies:

1. Set the Stage Before Play: Before engaging in group sexual activities, establish a dedicated time for discussion. This can include sharing desires, boundaries, and any specific fantasies or preferences. Setting aside this time helps create a framework for open communication and ensures that everyone feels heard.

2. Use Clear Language: Encourage the use of clear and direct language when discussing boundaries and desires.   Avoid vague terms that can lead to misinterpretation.   For example, instead of saying "I'm okay with anything," be specific about what activities are enjoyable or off-limits.

3. Establish Check-Ins: During the encounter, incorporate regular check-ins to gauge comfort levels and ensure that all partners are enjoying the experience. Simple questions like "How are you feeling?" or "Is this okay for you?" can help maintain an open dialogue and address any concerns promptly.

4. Utilize Non-Verbal Cues: While verbal communication is crucial, non-verbal cues can also play a significant role in group dynamics. Encourage participants to establish signals (e.g., a raised hand or specific gestures) to indicate comfort or discomfort without disrupting the flow of the encounter.

5. Foster a Safe Environment: Create a safe space for communication by emphasizing the importance of respect and confidentiality. Reassure partners that their feelings and boundaries will be honored, which can help reduce anxiety around expressing needs.

6. Practice Active Listening: Encourage active listening among participants. This involves fully focusing on the speaker, acknowledging their feelings, and responding thoughtfully.   Active listening fosters empathy and understanding, which can enhance group dynamics.

7. Address Power Dynamics: Be mindful of power dynamics within the group. Encourage all participants to voice their opinions and desires, regardless of their perceived status.   This can help create a more equitable environment where everyone feels empowered to communicate.

8. Utilize Technology: In some cases, technology can facilitate communication. Consider using group messaging apps or anonymous feedback tools to allow participants to share their thoughts and feelings without direct confrontation.

Examples of Effective Communication

To illustrate the importance of maintaining open lines of communication, consider the following scenarios:

Scenario 1: Pre-Encounter Discussion   Before a group encounter, participants gather to discuss their boundaries.   One partner expresses a desire to explore BDSM elements, while another is uncomfortable with that.   By openly discussing these preferences, the group can establish clear boundaries and create a plan that respects everyone's comfort levels.

Scenario 2: In-the-Moment Check-In   During a group encounter, one partner notices that another seems less engaged. They pause the action and ask, "Are you okay? Do you want to try something different?" This simple check-in allows the disengaged partner to express their feelings and ensures that everyone is enjoying the experience.

Scenario 3: Post-Encounter Reflection   After a group encounter, participants gather for a debriefing session. They share what they enjoyed, what could be improved, and any emotional reactions they experienced. This reflective practice fosters emotional intimacy and helps participants learn from the experience.

Conclusion

Maintaining open lines of communication with group partners is essential for creating a safe, pleasurable, and fulfilling sexual experience.   By prioritizing clear dialogue, addressing challenges, and implementing effective strategies, participants can enhance their group encounters and deepen their connections with one another.   Remember, communication is not just a tool for consent; it is a pathway to shared pleasure and intimacy in the beautiful tapestry of group sexual exploration.

Addressing Jealousy, Insecurity, and Envy in Group Dynamics

In the realm of group sexual encounters, feelings of jealousy, insecurity, and envy can emerge, often complicating what is meant to be a liberating and pleasurable experience. Recognizing these emotions and addressing them head-on is crucial for maintaining a positive atmosphere and ensuring that all participants feel valued and secure.

Understanding the Roots of Jealousy and Insecurity

Jealousy and insecurity often stem from various sources, including personal insecurities, past experiences, and societal conditioning. The fear of inadequacy or the belief that one's partner may find someone else more attractive or fulfilling can lead to heightened emotional responses.

$$J = f(P, E, S) \tag{18}$$

Where:

+ J represents the level of jealousy experienced,

+ P is the individual's personal insecurities,

+ E denotes past emotional experiences,

+ S symbolizes societal influences and norms.

Recognizing that these feelings are often rooted in personal narratives can help individuals contextualize their emotions and reduce the intensity of their reactions.

Open Communication: The Key to Mitigating Negative Emotions

Creating an environment where open communication is encouraged is paramount. Discussing fears and insecurities before engaging in group dynamics can foster understanding and empathy among participants. Here are some strategies to facilitate effective communication:

+ **Pre-Encounter Discussions**: Before any group play, gather all participants to discuss their feelings, boundaries, and any insecurities they may have. This sets a foundation of trust and openness.

+ **Check-Ins During Play**: Encourage participants to check in with one another during the encounter. Simple questions like, "How are you feeling?" can help address any arising discomfort before it escalates.

+ **Post-Encounter Debriefs**: After the experience, hold a debriefing session to discuss what went well and what could be improved. This reinforces the idea that everyone's feelings are valid and heard.

Reframing Jealousy as a Source of Growth

Instead of viewing jealousy solely as a negative emotion, it can be reframed as an opportunity for personal growth and deeper connection. For instance, recognizing feelings of jealousy can prompt individuals to explore their self-worth and enhance their communication skills.

$$G = J \cdot C \tag{19}$$

Where:

+ G represents personal growth,

+ J is the level of jealousy experienced,

+ C denotes the commitment to communication.

As individuals work through their feelings, they can emerge with a stronger sense of self and improved relationships with their partners.

Practicing Empathy and Compersion

Empathy is a powerful tool in addressing jealousy and insecurity. By actively trying to understand and share the feelings of others, participants can cultivate a supportive environment. Additionally, the concept of compersion—the joy derived from seeing one's partner experience pleasure with others—can be a transformative approach.

+ **Empathy Exercises**: Engage in exercises that allow participants to express their feelings and listen to others without judgment. For example, using "I feel" statements can help articulate emotions without assigning blame.

+ **Cultivating Compersion**: Encourage participants to celebrate each other's pleasure. This can be practiced through verbal affirmations or physical gestures that acknowledge and appreciate the enjoyment of others.

Navigating Group Dynamics: Strategies for Success

Understanding the dynamics of the group is essential in managing feelings of jealousy and insecurity. Here are some strategies to navigate these dynamics effectively:

+ **Set Clear Expectations**: Establishing clear expectations about the encounter can help mitigate misunderstandings and reduce feelings of inadequacy.

+ **Balance Attention**: Ensure that all participants feel included and valued. This can be achieved by rotating partners or ensuring that everyone has a chance to engage with each other.

+ **Encourage Individual Time**: Allow for moments where individuals can connect one-on-one, fostering intimacy and reducing feelings of competition.

Conclusion

Addressing jealousy, insecurity, and envy within group dynamics requires intentionality, empathy, and open communication. By fostering an environment of trust and support, participants can navigate these complex emotions, enhancing their collective experience. Remember, it's not about eliminating these feelings but learning to understand and manage them, transforming potential obstacles into opportunities for connection and growth. Embrace the journey together, and let your shared pleasure flourish.

Establishing Consent Protocols and Safe Words in Group Play

In the realm of group sexual encounters, establishing clear consent protocols and safe words is paramount to ensuring a safe, enjoyable, and fulfilling experience for all participants. Consent is not merely a checkbox; it is an ongoing dialogue that fosters trust, respect, and emotional safety. This section delves into the importance of consent protocols, how to establish them effectively, and the role of safe words in group dynamics.

The Importance of Consent Protocols

Consent protocols serve as the foundation for any sexual encounter, particularly in group settings where the dynamics can become more complex. Understanding that consent is a fluid and dynamic process rather than a one-time agreement is crucial. It is essential to recognize that consent must be:

- **Informed:** All participants should have a clear understanding of what activities will take place, including potential risks and boundaries.

- **Freely Given:** Consent should be given without coercion, manipulation, or pressure. Each participant must feel empowered to say "no" at any time.

- **Revocable:** Consent can be withdrawn at any moment. Participants should feel safe to change their minds without fear of repercussions.

- **Enthusiastic:** Consent should be expressed with enthusiasm. A lack of resistance does not equate to consent.

Establishing Consent Protocols

Creating a framework for consent involves open communication and negotiation before engaging in sexual activities. Here are steps to establish effective consent protocols:

1. **Pre-Encounter Discussions:** Before any group sexual activity, gather all participants to discuss boundaries, desires, and limits. This is the time to express individual preferences and establish what is off-limits. Use open-ended questions to facilitate dialogue, such as:

   "What are you excited to explore?"
   "Are there any hard limits we should be aware of?"

2. **Create a Consent Checklist:** Consider developing a checklist that outlines various activities and allows participants to indicate their comfort levels. This can help clarify what everyone is interested in and what should be avoided.

3. **Establish Safe Words:** Safe words are critical in group scenarios, providing a way for participants to communicate their comfort levels effectively. Choose simple, easily remembered words that are unlikely to be used in casual conversation. Common examples include:

   + **Red:** Stop all activities immediately.

   + **Yellow:** Slow down or check in; the participant is feeling unsure but not necessarily wanting to stop.

   + **Green:** Everything is okay; continue as planned.

4. **Check-Ins During Play:** Encourage regular check-ins throughout the encounter. This can be as simple as asking, "How is everyone feeling?" or "Are we still good to continue?" This practice reinforces the importance of consent and ensures that everyone remains comfortable.

5. **Post-Encounter Debrief:** After the encounter, hold a debriefing session where participants can share their experiences, feelings, and any concerns. This is an opportunity to discuss what went well and what could be improved for future encounters.

Addressing Potential Problems

Despite the best intentions, misunderstandings can occur. It's vital to be prepared for potential issues related to consent in group settings:

- **Miscommunication:** Ensure that everyone understands the established protocols. Miscommunication can lead to discomfort or breaches of consent.

- **Overstepping Boundaries:** Participants may inadvertently push boundaries if they are not clearly communicated. Reinforcing the importance of safe words can help mitigate this risk.

- **Emotional Reactions:** Group dynamics can elicit strong emotional responses. Be prepared to address feelings of jealousy, insecurity, or discomfort that may arise during or after the encounter.

Examples of Consent in Action

Consider the following scenarios to illustrate the importance of consent protocols and safe words:

- **Scenario 1:** During a group encounter, one participant feels overwhelmed and uses the safe word "Red." All activities stop immediately, and the group checks in with the participant to ensure their emotional and physical safety.

- **Scenario 2:** A participant expresses a desire to try a new activity during the encounter. They pause to check in with others, ensuring everyone is comfortable before proceeding. This demonstrates respect for group dynamics and individual boundaries.

- **Scenario 3:** After a group play session, participants gather for a debrief. One person shares that they felt uncomfortable with a specific activity, prompting a discussion on how to improve communication and consent for future encounters.

Conclusion

Establishing consent protocols and safe words is not merely a formality; it is a vital aspect of creating a safe and pleasurable environment in group sexual encounters. By prioritizing clear communication, mutual respect, and emotional safety, participants can enhance their experiences and foster deeper connections. Remember, consent is an ongoing conversation, and everyone involved should feel empowered to express their needs and boundaries at all times.

> "Consent is the foundation of any intimate encounter. In group settings, it becomes even more essential to ensure that everyone feels safe, respected, and heard."

Navigating Consent Negotiations and Giving/Receiving Feedback

In the realm of group sexual encounters, consent is not merely a checkbox to be ticked off; it is a dynamic, ongoing process that requires attention, communication, and mutual respect. The negotiation of consent and the practice of giving and receiving feedback are essential components that enhance the safety and pleasure of all participants involved. This section will explore the theoretical foundations of consent negotiation, common challenges, and practical strategies for effective communication.

Theoretical Foundations of Consent

Consent is rooted in the principles of autonomy and respect for individual agency. According to the *Consent Model*, consent must be:

- **Informed:** All parties should have a clear understanding of what they are consenting to, including the activities involved, potential risks, and boundaries.

- **Freely Given:** Consent must be given voluntarily without coercion or manipulation.

- **Reversible:** Anyone can withdraw their consent at any time, and this decision must be respected.

- **Enthusiastic:** Consent should be expressed with eagerness and excitement, rather than reluctance or obligation.

These principles create a framework for navigating consent in group scenarios, ensuring that every participant feels empowered and respected.

Common Challenges in Consent Negotiation

Navigating consent in group settings can present unique challenges, including:

- **Miscommunication:** In larger groups, messages can become muddled, leading to misunderstandings about boundaries and desires.

- **Power Dynamics:** Hierarchical structures or pre-existing relationships can complicate consent, as individuals may feel pressured to conform to the desires of more dominant partners.

- **Fear of Rejection:** Participants may hesitate to express their true desires or boundaries due to fears of judgment or rejection from others.

- **Emotional Vulnerability:** The intimacy of sexual encounters can heighten emotional sensitivities, making it difficult for individuals to voice concerns or feedback.

Addressing these challenges requires intentionality and a commitment to open communication.

Strategies for Navigating Consent Negotiations

1. **Pre-Encounter Discussions:** Before engaging in group play, hold a discussion with all participants to establish boundaries, desires, and limits. Use open-ended questions to facilitate dialogue, such as:

> "What are your boundaries when it comes to physical touch?"

and

> "Are there any specific activities you are particularly excited about or wish to avoid?"

This conversation sets the stage for mutual understanding and respect.

2. **Use of Consent Tools:** Implementing tools such as a *consent checklist* or *negotiation scripts* can help clarify desires and boundaries. A checklist might include options for activities, safe words, and limits. This structured approach can alleviate anxiety and ensure that everyone's preferences are acknowledged.

3. **Active Listening:** Foster an environment of active listening where participants feel heard and valued. Encourage the use of reflective listening techniques, such as paraphrasing what someone has said to confirm understanding. For example:

"So, what I hear you saying is that you're comfortable with kissing but prefer to avoid any penetration. Is that correct?"

4. **Establishing Safe Words:** Safe words provide a clear and immediate way to communicate discomfort or the need to pause an activity. Agree on a simple system, such as a traffic light model where:

+ **Green:** Everything is good; keep going.

+ **Yellow:** Slow down or check in.

+ **Red:** Stop immediately.

5. **Feedback Loops:** Create opportunities for feedback during and after encounters. Encourage participants to share their experiences and feelings, which can enhance emotional intimacy and improve future encounters. Questions to prompt feedback could include:

"How did you feel about our interactions during the encounter?"

and

"Is there anything you would like to adjust for next time?"

6. **Post-Encounter Check-Ins:** After the experience, take time to check in with each other. This not only reinforces emotional connections but also provides a space to discuss what went well and what could be improved. This practice nurtures ongoing trust and communication.

Examples of Effective Consent Negotiation

Consider the following scenario:

A group of four individuals is preparing for a weekend retreat that includes sexual exploration. During their pre-encounter discussion, they use a consent checklist to outline their interests and boundaries. One participant expresses a desire to explore BDSM, while another is uncomfortable with that dynamic. They agree to establish a safe word and decide that any BDSM activities will only occur if all participants are enthusiastic about it.

During the encounter, one individual feels overwhelmed and uses the safe word. The group immediately stops and checks in, allowing the person to express their feelings and adjust the activities accordingly. Afterward, they engage in a feedback loop, discussing what each person enjoyed and what could be improved for future encounters.

This scenario illustrates how effective consent negotiation and feedback can enhance the experience for everyone involved.

Conclusion

Navigating consent negotiations and giving/receiving feedback in group sexual encounters is essential for fostering a safe and pleasurable environment. By prioritizing open communication, actively listening, and respecting individual boundaries, participants can create a foundation of trust and mutual respect. Remember, consent is an ongoing conversation, and the commitment to maintaining it enhances the overall experience for everyone involved. Embrace the process, and let it empower your exploration of pleasure in group settings.

Handling Conflict and Resolving Disagreements in Group Scenarios

In any group sexual encounter, the potential for conflict and disagreement is an inherent part of the experience. Navigating these situations with grace and respect is essential for maintaining a safe and pleasurable environment. This section will explore effective strategies for handling conflict and resolving disagreements in group scenarios, ensuring that all participants feel valued and heard.

Understanding Conflict in Group Dynamics

Conflict can arise from various sources, including miscommunication, differing expectations, and emotional triggers. It is crucial to recognize that conflict is not inherently negative; rather, it can be an opportunity for growth and deeper understanding among participants. According to the *Conflict Resolution Theory*, addressing issues head-on can lead to more robust relationships and enhanced emotional intimacy.

Common Sources of Conflict

1. **Miscommunication**: Misunderstandings can occur when partners fail to express their desires or boundaries clearly. For instance, if one partner assumes that everyone is comfortable with a particular activity without verifying consent, it can lead to feelings of violation and resentment.

2. **Differing Expectations**: Participants may enter a group scenario with varying expectations about what the encounter will entail. For example, one person might view the encounter as a casual experience, while another may seek a deeper emotional connection. This discrepancy can lead to disappointment and conflict.

3. **Emotional Triggers**: Group dynamics can evoke past traumas or insecurities, leading to reactions that may seem disproportionate to the situation at hand. For instance, feelings of jealousy or inadequacy can surface if one partner receives more attention than another.

Strategies for Conflict Resolution

To effectively handle conflicts in group scenarios, consider the following strategies:

1. Open Communication   Encourage an environment where all participants feel safe expressing their thoughts and feelings. Utilize *active listening* techniques, which involve fully concentrating on what is being said rather than formulating a response while the other person is speaking. This fosters understanding and validates each person's perspective.

2. Establish Ground Rules   Prior to engaging in group play, establish clear ground rules regarding communication and conflict resolution. For example, agree on a safe word or signal that any participant can use to pause the encounter if they feel uncomfortable or need to address an issue. This proactive approach can prevent misunderstandings and provide a framework for resolving conflicts.

3. Use "I" Statements   When discussing conflicts, encourage participants to use "I" statements to express their feelings without placing blame. For instance, instead of saying, "You made me uncomfortable," one might say, "I felt uncomfortable when the activity shifted without checking in with me." This technique helps to reduce defensiveness and encourages a more constructive dialogue.

4. Take a Break if Needed   If tensions rise, it may be beneficial to take a short break from the encounter. This pause allows participants to gather their thoughts, calm their emotions, and reflect on the situation. During this time, individuals can also engage in self-soothing techniques, such as deep breathing or mindfulness exercises.

5. Facilitate a Group Discussion   If a conflict persists, facilitate a group discussion to address the issue collectively. Ensure that each person has the opportunity to share their perspective without interruption. Utilize a mediator if necessary, someone who can help guide the conversation and keep it focused on resolution rather than blame.

6. Focus on Solutions Encourage participants to shift their focus from the problem to potential solutions. Brainstorming together can foster collaboration and strengthen group dynamics. For example, if a participant feels neglected, the group might agree to implement a rotation system for attention during the encounter.

After the Conflict: Reflection and Growth

After a conflict has been resolved, it is essential to reflect on the experience. Encourage participants to discuss what they learned from the situation and how they can apply these insights in future encounters. This reflection can enhance emotional intimacy and reinforce the importance of communication and consent within the group.

Example Scenario

Consider a situation where two participants, Alex and Jamie, disagree about the level of physical intimacy they are comfortable with during a group encounter. Alex feels pressured to engage in more intimate acts, while Jamie prefers to take things slowly.

1. **Identify the Conflict**: Alex expresses discomfort with the pace of the encounter, while Jamie feels overwhelmed by the pressure to perform.

2. **Open Communication**: They take a moment to step aside and communicate their feelings using "I" statements.

3. **Establish Ground Rules**: They agree to pause the encounter and check in with each other regularly to ensure both feel comfortable.

4. **Facilitate a Group Discussion**: They involve the other participants to discuss the pace of the encounter and agree to a more gradual approach.

5. **Reflection**: After the encounter, Alex and Jamie discuss what worked well and what could be improved for next time, reinforcing their communication skills and emotional connection.

Conclusion

Handling conflict and resolving disagreements in group scenarios requires a commitment to open communication, empathy, and respect. By fostering an environment where all participants feel safe to express their needs and concerns, groups can navigate conflicts effectively and enhance their collective experience. Remember, conflict is a natural part of any relationship; how you handle it can ultimately strengthen the bonds between partners and lead to greater satisfaction in group encounters.

Practicing Active Listening and Empathy in Group Settings

In the context of group sexual encounters, the dynamics of communication can significantly influence the overall experience. Practicing active listening and empathy is crucial for fostering a safe and pleasurable environment. This section delves into the theoretical foundations of active listening, the importance of empathy, common challenges faced in group settings, and practical strategies to enhance these skills.

Theoretical Foundations of Active Listening

Active listening is a communication technique that involves fully concentrating, understanding, responding, and remembering what is being said. According to Carl Rogers, a prominent psychologist, active listening is essential for creating a supportive environment where individuals feel heard and valued. It encompasses several key components:

- **Attention:** Giving full attention to the speaker without distractions.

- **Reflection:** Paraphrasing or summarizing what the speaker has said to confirm understanding.

- **Clarification:** Asking questions to gain deeper insight into the speaker's feelings and thoughts.

- **Validation:** Acknowledging the speaker's emotions and experiences as legitimate and important.

The Role of Empathy

Empathy, the ability to understand and share the feelings of another, is integral to effective communication in group scenarios. It allows participants to connect on a deeper emotional level, facilitating trust and intimacy. According to Brené Brown, empathy is a critical component of vulnerability, which can enhance emotional safety in sexual encounters.

Empathy can be broken down into three components:

+ **Cognitive Empathy:** The ability to understand another's perspective or mental state.

+ **Emotional Empathy:** The capacity to physically feel what another person is experiencing.

+ **Compassionate Empathy:** Going beyond understanding and feeling to actively support the other person.

Challenges in Group Settings

Despite the importance of active listening and empathy, several challenges can hinder effective communication in group sexual encounters:

+ **Distractions:** The presence of multiple stimuli can make it difficult to focus on individual conversations.

+ **Jealousy and Insecurity:** Participants may struggle to listen actively if they are preoccupied with feelings of jealousy or self-doubt.

+ **Misinterpretation:** Non-verbal cues can be easily misread in a group setting, leading to misunderstandings.

+ **Power Dynamics:** Imbalances in power or status among group members can inhibit open communication.

Practical Strategies for Enhancing Active Listening and Empathy

To overcome these challenges, participants can adopt several practical strategies:

1. **Create a Safe Space:** Establish ground rules that encourage open dialogue and respect for each person's voice. This can include agreeing to speak one at a time and using "I" statements to express feelings.

2. **Practice Mindfulness:** Engage in mindfulness exercises before group encounters to enhance focus and presence. Techniques such as deep breathing can help participants remain calm and attentive during discussions.

3. **Use Reflective Listening:** When someone shares their thoughts or feelings, practice reflective listening by paraphrasing their statements. For example, if a partner expresses concern about feeling left out, respond with, "It sounds like you're worried about not being included in the experience."

4. **Encourage Vulnerability:** Create an environment where participants feel safe to express their insecurities and desires. This can be facilitated through sharing personal stories or discussing fantasies in a non-judgmental way.

5. **Implement Check-Ins:** Regularly pause during the encounter to check in with all participants about their feelings and comfort levels. This can help address any issues before they escalate.

6. **Practice Empathy Exercises:** Engage in activities that promote empathy, such as role-playing or perspective-taking exercises, where participants switch roles to understand each other's experiences better.

Examples of Active Listening and Empathy in Action

Consider a scenario where a participant expresses discomfort with a particular activity. An active listener might respond by saying, "I hear that you're feeling uncomfortable with this. Can you share more about what specifically is bothering you?" This approach validates the speaker's feelings and encourages open communication.

In another instance, if someone shares their excitement about a new fantasy they want to explore, an empathetic response could be, "That sounds really exciting! I'm curious to hear more about what that looks like for you." This not only acknowledges their enthusiasm but also invites further discussion, deepening the emotional connection.

Conclusion

Practicing active listening and empathy in group sexual encounters is essential for creating a pleasurable and safe environment. By understanding the theoretical foundations, recognizing challenges, and implementing practical strategies, participants can enhance their communication skills. This will not only enrich their individual experiences but also strengthen the connections within the group, ultimately leading to more fulfilling and enjoyable encounters.

Emotional Support and Aftercare in Group Sexual Encounters

In the realm of group sexual encounters, emotional support and aftercare are crucial components that can significantly enhance the overall experience. After engaging in intimate activities, participants may experience a variety of emotions, ranging from exhilaration to vulnerability. This section will explore the importance of emotional support and aftercare, offering practical strategies to navigate these dynamics effectively.

Understanding the Importance of Aftercare

Aftercare refers to the practices and interactions that occur following a sexual encounter, especially one that involves heightened emotional and physical intensity. It serves several purposes:

1. **Emotional Regulation**: Aftercare helps individuals process their feelings post-encounter. This is particularly important in group settings where the emotional landscape can be complex due to the involvement of multiple partners. 2. **Reinforcement of Trust**: Engaging in aftercare can reinforce trust among participants. It signals that partners care for each other's well-being beyond the physical act.   3.   **Recovery and Reconnection**: Aftercare provides an opportunity for participants to reconnect and recover from the emotional and physical exertion of the encounter.

Common Emotional Responses

Participants in group sexual encounters may experience a range of emotions, including:

- **Euphoria**: The release of endorphins and oxytocin during sexual activity can lead to feelings of happiness and connection. - **Vulnerability**: Being exposed physically and emotionally can evoke feelings of vulnerability, especially in a group setting where dynamics can shift. - **Jealousy or Insecurity**: It's not uncommon for individuals to feel jealousy or insecurity when witnessing partners engaging with others. - **Post-Play Blues**: After the high of the encounter, some may feel a sense of letdown or sadness, known as post-play blues.

Recognizing these emotional responses is the first step in providing adequate support and aftercare.

Strategies for Effective Emotional Support

To ensure that all participants feel supported after a group encounter, consider the following strategies:

1. **Check-Ins**: Regularly check in with each participant after the encounter. Simple questions like "How are you feeling?" or "What was your favorite part?" can open the door for emotional expression. 2. **Active Listening**: Practice active listening by giving your full attention to the speaker. Validate their feelings and experiences without judgment. 3. **Group Debriefing**: Consider holding a group debriefing session where everyone can share their thoughts and feelings about the encounter. This can foster a sense of community and shared experience. 4. **Physical Affection**: Engage in physical aftercare practices such as cuddling, holding hands, or gentle touch. This can help soothe any lingering anxiety and reinforce emotional bonds. 5. **Affirmation and Reassurance**: Offer words of affirmation and reassurance to help alleviate feelings of insecurity. Remind participants of their desirability and worthiness.

Creating a Safe Space for Aftercare

Creating a safe and welcoming environment for aftercare is essential. Here are some tips for fostering such an atmosphere:

- **Comfortable Setting**: Ensure the space is comfortable and conducive to relaxation. Soft lighting, cozy blankets, and soothing music can enhance the aftercare experience. - **Establish Boundaries**: Before engaging in aftercare, establish boundaries regarding what participants are comfortable with in terms of physical touch and emotional sharing. - **Respect Individual Needs**: Recognize that each individual may have different needs regarding aftercare. Some may prefer solitude, while others may seek companionship. Be attentive to these preferences.

Examples of Aftercare Practices

Here are some practical examples of aftercare practices that can be beneficial in group scenarios:

- **Hydration and Snacks**: Providing water and light snacks can help replenish energy levels and foster a sense of care and consideration. - **Guided Relaxation**: Engage in guided relaxation techniques or breathing exercises to help participants ground themselves after the encounter. - **Journaling**: Encourage participants to journal their thoughts and feelings about the experience. This can be a therapeutic way to process emotions and reflect on personal growth. - **Follow-Up Communication**: After the encounter, maintain communication with all participants. A simple message expressing gratitude or checking in can go a long way in reinforcing emotional connections.

Addressing Challenges in Aftercare

While aftercare is vital, it can also present challenges. Some common issues include:
- **Miscommunication**: Misunderstandings about aftercare needs can lead to feelings of neglect or resentment. Clear communication is essential. - **Overwhelm**: Some individuals may feel overwhelmed by the emotional intensity of the encounter and may need time alone rather than immediate interaction. - **Differing Needs**: Each participant may have different aftercare needs, which can complicate the process. It's important to be flexible and accommodating.

To address these challenges, encourage open dialogue about aftercare preferences before engaging in group play. This proactive approach can help set expectations and reduce misunderstandings.

Conclusion

Emotional support and aftercare are essential components of group sexual encounters. By prioritizing these practices, participants can foster deeper connections, enhance emotional well-being, and ensure a fulfilling experience for everyone involved. Remember, the journey doesn't end with the act; it continues through the care and consideration shown to one another in the aftermath. Embrace the power of aftercare, and let it be a celebration of intimacy, trust, and shared pleasure.

Maintaining Group Dynamics and Reevaluating Group Agreements

In group sexual encounters, maintaining healthy dynamics and periodically reevaluating group agreements is essential for fostering a safe, enjoyable, and consensual environment. As the dynamics of the group shift—whether due to new participants, changing relationships, or evolving desires—it's crucial to engage in ongoing communication and reflection. This section will explore the theoretical underpinnings of group dynamics, common challenges that may arise, and practical strategies for ensuring that all participants feel respected and fulfilled.

Theoretical Framework of Group Dynamics

Group dynamics refer to the behavioral and psychological processes that occur within a social group. According to Tuckman's stages of group development, groups typically progress through five stages: forming, storming, norming, performing, and adjourning [?]. Understanding these stages can help participants recognize where their group stands and what adjustments may be necessary.

1. **Forming:** Initial interactions where members get to know each other and establish group norms. 2. **Storming:** Conflicts may arise as individuals assert their opinions and desires, leading to potential misunderstandings. 3. **Norming:** The group begins to establish a sense of cohesion and shared understanding, which is crucial for consent and boundaries. 4. **Performing:** The group functions effectively, and members feel comfortable expressing their needs and desires. 5. **Adjourning:** The group disbands, which may require reflection on the experience and closure for participants.

Understanding these stages can help participants navigate their experiences more effectively and adapt their agreements as necessary.

Common Challenges in Group Dynamics

While engaging in group sexual encounters can be exhilarating, it may also present unique challenges that can disrupt group dynamics. Some common issues include:

- **Jealousy and Insecurity:** Feelings of jealousy can arise, particularly if one partner appears to be receiving more attention or pleasure. This can lead to tension and discomfort among participants. - **Miscommunication:** Assumptions about desires and boundaries can lead to misunderstandings. It is essential to communicate openly and clearly about what each person wants and needs. - **Power Imbalances:** Differences in experience, confidence, or social status can create power dynamics that may impact group interactions. Recognizing and addressing these imbalances is crucial for maintaining a healthy environment. - **Evolving Desires:** As individuals engage in group play, their desires and boundaries may shift. Regular check-ins can help ensure that everyone is still comfortable and enthusiastic about the activities taking place.

Strategies for Maintaining Group Dynamics

To foster positive group dynamics and ensure that all participants feel valued and respected, consider the following strategies:

+ **Regular Check-Ins:** Schedule periodic check-ins during and after group encounters to discuss feelings, experiences, and any concerns that may arise. This can help participants feel heard and supported.

+ **Revisiting Agreements:** Encourage participants to revisit and revise group agreements as needed. This could involve discussing boundaries, consent protocols, and any new desires or limits that may have emerged.

+ **Establishing Safe Words:** Utilize safe words or signals that participants can use to pause or stop activities if they feel uncomfortable. This empowers individuals to advocate for their needs and reinforces a culture of consent.

+ **Encouraging Open Communication:** Foster an environment where all participants feel comfortable expressing their feelings and desires. This can be achieved through active listening and creating a non-judgmental space for sharing.

+ **Addressing Issues Promptly:** If conflicts or concerns arise, address them as soon as possible to prevent escalation. Openly discussing issues can help restore harmony and trust within the group.

Example Scenario

Consider a group of four friends who regularly engage in group sexual encounters. After a particularly intense session, one participant expresses feeling overlooked as others seemed to connect more intimately. Instead of ignoring this discomfort, the group decides to hold a check-in.

During the check-in, they discuss how everyone felt during the encounter, allowing the concerned participant to voice their feelings. The group acknowledges the concern and agrees to adjust their approach in future sessions, ensuring that everyone receives equal attention and pleasure.

This scenario illustrates the importance of maintaining open lines of communication and the willingness to adapt agreements to better meet the needs of all participants.

Conclusion

Maintaining group dynamics and reevaluating group agreements is an ongoing process that requires commitment, empathy, and open communication. By recognizing the complexities of group interactions and actively addressing challenges, participants can create a fulfilling and pleasurable environment where everyone feels empowered to explore their desires. Regular check-ins, revisiting agreements, and fostering a culture of consent are vital components of this process, ensuring that group sexual encounters remain enjoyable and enriching for all involved.

Recognizing and Respecting Individual Autonomy in Group Play

In the context of group sexual encounters, recognizing and respecting individual autonomy is paramount. Autonomy refers to the capacity to make informed, uncoerced decisions about one's own body and sexual experiences. In group settings, where multiple desires, boundaries, and dynamics intersect, it becomes essential to honor each participant's right to agency. This section will explore the theoretical underpinnings of autonomy, the challenges it presents in group contexts, and practical strategies to ensure that every individual feels empowered and respected.

Theoretical Framework of Autonomy

Autonomy is rooted in ethical theories that prioritize individual rights and self-determination. According to Kantian ethics, individuals should be treated as ends in themselves, not merely as means to an end. This principle applies directly to sexual encounters, where each person's desires and boundaries must be acknowledged and respected. Furthermore, feminist ethics emphasizes the importance of consent and mutual respect in sexual relationships, advocating for an environment where all participants feel safe to express their needs and limits.

Challenges to Autonomy in Group Scenarios

Despite the theoretical importance of autonomy, various challenges can impede its realization in group sexual encounters:

- **Power Dynamics:** In groups, power imbalances can emerge, particularly if one or more individuals hold more influence or authority. This can lead to coercion, whether overt or subtle, undermining the autonomy of less dominant participants.

- **Peer Pressure:** The desire to fit in or please others can pressure individuals to override their own boundaries. This is particularly acute in group scenarios where the social dynamics are fluid and complex.

+ **Miscommunication:** In the heat of the moment, individuals may struggle to articulate their needs or limits, leading to misunderstandings that can compromise autonomy.

+ **Emotional Vulnerability:** Group settings can amplify feelings of insecurity or jealousy, which may lead individuals to suppress their true desires to avoid conflict or discomfort.

Strategies for Upholding Autonomy

To foster an environment that respects individual autonomy, consider implementing the following strategies:

1. **Clear Communication:** Establish open lines of communication before and during the encounter. Encourage participants to express their boundaries, desires, and any concerns they may have. Utilize tools such as "yes/no/maybe" lists to facilitate discussions about preferences and limits.

2. **Consent Check-Ins:** Regularly check in with all participants to ensure that everyone feels comfortable and respected. This can be done verbally or through non-verbal cues, allowing individuals to express their feelings without pressure.

3. **Empowering Language:** Use language that affirms individual autonomy. Phrases like "What do you want?" or "How does that feel for you?" can empower participants to voice their needs and desires.

4. **Establishing Safe Words:** Create a system of safe words or signals that anyone can use to pause or stop the encounter if they feel uncomfortable. This reinforces the idea that everyone has the right to change their mind at any time.

5. **Addressing Power Imbalances:** Be mindful of the dynamics at play within the group. If certain individuals appear to dominate the conversation or decision-making, actively encourage quieter members to share their thoughts and feelings.

6. **Aftercare and Debriefing:** After the encounter, engage in a debriefing session where participants can discuss their experiences, feelings, and any issues that arose. This process not only validates individual experiences but also fosters a sense of community and support.

Examples of Respecting Autonomy

Consider the following scenarios to illustrate how respecting autonomy can manifest in group sexual encounters:

> **Example**
>
> During a group play session, one participant expresses discomfort with a particular activity. The group pauses immediately, and the facilitator asks if anyone else shares similar feelings. After a brief discussion, the group collectively agrees to pivot to a different activity, ensuring everyone's comfort and enjoyment.

> **Example**
>
> In another scenario, a participant shares a fantasy that involves a specific role-play. The group engages in a discussion about this fantasy, allowing everyone to voice their comfort levels and boundaries. Some members express interest, while others decline. The individual is encouraged to explore their fantasy with willing partners, reinforcing their autonomy while respecting the limits of others.

Conclusion

Recognizing and respecting individual autonomy in group sexual encounters is essential for creating a safe, pleasurable, and empowering environment. By understanding the theoretical foundations of autonomy, addressing the challenges that arise, and implementing clear strategies for communication and consent, participants can ensure that everyone's desires and boundaries are honored. Ultimately, fostering an atmosphere of respect and empowerment not only enhances individual experiences but also enriches the collective dynamic of the group, leading to deeper connections and more fulfilling encounters.

Riding the Wave: Techniques for Multiple Orgasms in Group Scenarios

Building Arousal and Sexual Energy in Group Settings

Group Foreplay Techniques: Teasing, Touching, and Kissing

Group foreplay is an essential component of maximizing pleasure in any sexual encounter, particularly in group scenarios where the dynamics can be both exciting and complex. This section will explore various techniques for teasing, touching, and kissing that can enhance arousal and create a deeper connection among participants.

The Importance of Foreplay in Group Settings

Foreplay serves multiple purposes in group sexual encounters. It helps to build anticipation, enhances intimacy, and allows individuals to gauge each other's comfort levels and desires. Engaging in foreplay can also facilitate communication and consent, as participants express their preferences and boundaries through touch and interaction.

$$E = \sum_{i=1}^{n} T_i \tag{20}$$

Where E is the overall enjoyment, and T_i represents the teasing and touching techniques employed by each participant i. The more techniques utilized, the greater the potential for heightened arousal and pleasure.

Teasing Techniques

Teasing is a powerful tool in foreplay that can build tension and excitement. Here are some effective teasing techniques for group encounters:

- **Verbal Teasing:** Use suggestive language and playful banter to create a charged atmosphere. Complimenting each other's bodies, whispering fantasies, or playfully challenging one another can heighten anticipation.

- **Visual Teasing:** Encourage participants to dress in a way that highlights their bodies, or engage in playful stripteases. This not only excites the group but also fosters confidence and body positivity.

- **Physical Teasing:** Lightly touch or brush against others without fully engaging. For example, a gentle graze of fingers along an arm or a playful poke can be electrifying. The key is to maintain an element of surprise and restraint.

Touching Techniques

Touching is a fundamental aspect of foreplay that deepens physical connection. Here are some techniques to explore:

- **Exploratory Touching:** Encourage participants to explore each other's bodies in a consensual manner. This could involve tracing fingers along curves, exploring erogenous zones, or discovering sensitive areas that elicit pleasure.

- **Layered Touching:** Utilize multiple points of contact. For example, one partner can kiss while another caresses the body. This layered approach can create a symphony of sensations and amplify arousal.

- **Synchronizing Touch:** Coordinate touches among participants. For instance, if one person is kissing another, others can join in by touching the recipient's body simultaneously, creating a harmonious experience that enhances connection.

Kissing Techniques

Kissing is an intimate act that can significantly enhance foreplay. Here are some techniques to incorporate:

- **Group Kissing:** Encourage a circle where participants can kiss each other in a sequence. This not only spreads affection but also creates a playful and inclusive atmosphere.

- **Kissing Variations:** Experiment with different types of kisses—soft pecks, deep passionate kisses, or playful nibbles. Each variation can evoke different emotions and levels of arousal.

- **Kissing Games:** Introduce playful games that involve kissing, such as "Truth or Dare," where dares involve kissing a specific participant or part of their body. This can break the ice and encourage laughter and fun.

Addressing Common Challenges

While engaging in group foreplay, participants may encounter challenges such as insecurity, jealousy, or miscommunication. Here are strategies to navigate these issues:

- **Open Communication:** Encourage participants to express their feelings and desires openly. Establishing a safe space for dialogue can help mitigate insecurities and foster trust.

- **Check-Ins:** Regularly check in with one another to ensure everyone is comfortable and enjoying themselves. This can be as simple as asking, "How does this feel for you?" or "Are you comfortable with this?"

- **Respect Boundaries:** Always prioritize consent and respect personal boundaries. If someone expresses discomfort, it is crucial to immediately adjust the dynamics to ensure everyone feels safe and respected.

Conclusion

Incorporating effective teasing, touching, and kissing techniques into group foreplay can significantly enhance the overall experience, creating a pleasurable and intimate environment. By focusing on communication, consent, and exploration, participants can maximize their enjoyment and foster deeper connections. Embrace the power of foreplay as a means to ride the wave of pleasure together, setting the stage for an unforgettable group sexual encounter.

Utilizing Sensory Play and Erotic Massage in Group Scenarios

Sensory play and erotic massage can significantly enhance the pleasure and intimacy experienced in group sexual encounters. These practices not only heighten arousal but also foster deeper connections among participants. In this section, we will explore the theoretical foundations of sensory play and erotic massage, the potential challenges that may arise, and practical examples to help you integrate these elements into your group experiences.

Theoretical Foundations

Sensory play involves engaging the senses—touch, taste, sight, sound, and smell—to enhance erotic experiences. The theory behind sensory play is rooted in the understanding that our bodies respond to various stimuli, which can amplify pleasure and arousal. According to the *Dual Control Model* of sexual response proposed by Bancroft and Meston (2006), sexual arousal is influenced by both excitatory and inhibitory processes. Sensory play can stimulate the excitatory pathways, leading to increased arousal and pleasure.

Erotic massage, on the other hand, focuses on the intentional and pleasurable manipulation of the body. It can release physical tension, enhance relaxation, and promote emotional intimacy. Research indicates that touch can trigger the release of oxytocin, often referred to as the "love hormone," which fosters bonding and trust among participants (Uvnäs-Moberg, 1998).

Potential Challenges

While sensory play and erotic massage can enhance group encounters, several challenges may arise:

- **Consent and Comfort:** Not all participants may feel comfortable with certain types of touch or sensory experiences. It is crucial to establish clear communication about boundaries and preferences before engaging in these practices.

- **Overstimulation:** In a group setting, the multitude of sensations can lead to overstimulation for some individuals. It is important to remain attuned to each participant's responses and adjust activities accordingly.

- **Emotional Vulnerability:** Engaging in intimate touch can evoke strong emotions. Participants should be prepared for the possibility of unexpected feelings arising during sensory play and erotic massage.

Practical Examples

Here are several ways to incorporate sensory play and erotic massage into group scenarios:

1. Setting the Atmosphere Creating a conducive environment is essential for sensory play. Dim lighting, soft music, and comfortable surfaces can enhance the experience. Consider using scented candles or essential oils to stimulate the sense of smell, which can evoke feelings of relaxation and arousal.

2. Blindfolding Using blindfolds can heighten the experience of touch by removing the visual component. Participants can take turns being blindfolded while others explore their bodies with gentle caresses, teasing touches, or even varied objects like feathers or silk. This allows individuals to focus solely on their sense of touch and heightens anticipation.

3. Group Massage Circles Forming a massage circle where participants take turns giving and receiving erotic massages can foster intimacy and connection. Encourage participants to communicate their preferences regarding pressure, areas of focus, and techniques. This not only enhances pleasure but also builds trust and rapport among group members.

4. Sensory Stations Create sensory stations around the play area, each dedicated to a different sense. For example:

- **Touch Station:** Use various textures (e.g., feathers, silk, leather) for participants to explore on each other's bodies.

- **Taste Station:** Incorporate edible body products like flavored oils or chocolates that participants can use during massages or feeding each other.

- **Sound Station:** Play ambient sounds, erotic audiobooks, or music that participants can listen to while engaging in sensory play.

5. Temperature Play Incorporating temperature can add an exciting element to sensory play. Use warm oils for massage or introduce cold objects like ice cubes or chilled fruits. Participants can explore the contrasting sensations on each other's skin, enhancing arousal through surprise and anticipation.

6. Guided Sensory Experiences   Consider leading a guided sensory experience where participants are instructed to focus on their breath, tune into their bodies, and explore sensations slowly. This can include prompts for deep breathing, relaxing specific muscle groups, and encouraging participants to express their feelings and sensations verbally.

Conclusion

Utilizing sensory play and erotic massage in group scenarios can significantly amplify pleasure, intimacy, and emotional connection among participants.   By understanding the theoretical underpinnings, addressing potential challenges, and employing practical techniques, you can create a rich and fulfilling group sexual experience.   Remember, the key to successful sensory play lies in open communication, consent, and attentiveness to the needs and boundaries of all participants. Embrace the journey of exploration and connection, and let the waves of pleasure carry you and your partners to new heights of ecstasy.

Exploring Exhibitionism and Voyeurism in Group Encounters

Exhibitionism and voyeurism are two forms of sexual expression that can significantly enhance pleasure in group sexual encounters. Both practices involve a dynamic interplay of visibility and desire, allowing participants to explore their fantasies and boundaries in a consensual and safe environment.   Understanding these concepts is essential for maximizing pleasure and fostering a sense of connection among partners.

Defining Exhibitionism and Voyeurism

Exhibitionism is the act of exposing oneself sexually to others for the purpose of sexual arousal.   This can involve nudity, sexual acts, or other forms of sexual expression that are meant to be seen by others.   On the other hand, voyeurism refers to the enjoyment derived from watching others engage in sexual activities. Both exhibitionism and voyeurism can be practiced in various contexts, but they often find a particularly vibrant expression in group sexual encounters.

Theoretical Framework

The psychology behind exhibitionism and voyeurism can be understood through several theoretical lenses:

- **The Social Exchange Theory:** This theory posits that social behavior is the result of an exchange process aimed at maximizing benefits and minimizing costs. In the context of exhibitionism and voyeurism, participants may engage in these activities to gain pleasure, validation, or a sense of belonging within a group.

- **The Sexual Script Theory:** This framework suggests that sexual behavior is guided by socially constructed norms and scripts. Exhibitionists and voyeurs often navigate these scripts, negotiating their roles and expectations within the group dynamic.

- **The Concept of Consent:** Consent is paramount in both exhibitionism and voyeurism. Establishing clear boundaries and obtaining enthusiastic consent ensures that all participants feel safe and respected, enhancing the overall experience.

Benefits of Incorporating Exhibitionism and Voyeurism

Incorporating exhibitionism and voyeurism into group encounters can offer several benefits:

- **Heightened Arousal:** The thrill of being watched or watching others can significantly increase arousal levels, creating an electric atmosphere that enhances sexual experiences.

- **Enhanced Connection:** Sharing intimate moments in a group setting can foster a sense of community and connection among participants, deepening emotional bonds and trust.

- **Exploration of Fantasies:** Engaging in exhibitionism and voyeurism allows participants to explore their sexual fantasies in a safe and consensual environment, promoting sexual self-discovery and empowerment.

Navigating Challenges

While exhibitionism and voyeurism can enhance pleasure, they can also present challenges:

- **Insecurity and Body Image Issues:** Participants may feel vulnerable or insecure about their bodies. It is crucial to foster an environment of body positivity and acceptance, encouraging individuals to embrace their unique forms.

- **Consent and Boundaries:** Clear communication about consent and boundaries is essential. Participants should feel empowered to express their comfort levels and withdraw consent at any time.

- **Jealousy and Competition:** In group settings, feelings of jealousy or competition may arise. Establishing open communication can help address these feelings and promote a supportive environment.

Practical Examples

To effectively incorporate exhibitionism and voyeurism into group encounters, consider the following practical examples:

- **Setting the Scene:** Create an environment that encourages exhibitionism, such as dim lighting, mirrors, or a stage-like area where individuals can feel comfortable displaying their bodies or engaging in sexual acts.

- **Encouraging Participation:** Invite participants to take turns being the center of attention, allowing them to explore their exhibitionist desires while others engage in voyeuristic pleasure.

- **Role-Playing:** Incorporate role-playing scenarios that emphasize exhibitionism and voyeurism, such as a "peeping Tom" theme or a "striptease" performance, allowing participants to explore these dynamics in a playful manner.

Conclusion

Exploring exhibitionism and voyeurism in group encounters can lead to profound experiences of pleasure and connection. By understanding the theoretical frameworks, benefits, challenges, and practical applications of these practices, participants can create a rich and fulfilling sexual environment. Remember, the key to success lies in open communication, enthusiastic consent, and a commitment to fostering a safe and supportive atmosphere for all involved. Embrace the thrill of visibility and the joy of shared experiences, and let the waves of pleasure carry you to new heights of sexual fulfillment.

Incorporating Role-Playing and Fantasies in Group Play

Role-playing and the exploration of fantasies can significantly enhance the experience of group sexual encounters. By stepping into different roles or scenarios, participants can tap into their creativity, allowing for a deeper connection with their desires and the other individuals involved. This section will delve into the theory behind role-playing, address potential challenges, and provide practical examples to facilitate a fulfilling experience.

Theoretical Framework

Role-playing in sexual contexts can be understood through several psychological and sociological lenses. One prominent theory is the **Social Constructionist Theory**, which posits that sexual identities and practices are shaped by societal norms and personal experiences. This theory suggests that engaging in role-play allows individuals to explore identities that may be constrained by societal expectations, providing a safe space to experiment with different aspects of their sexuality.

Additionally, **Fantasy Theory** emphasizes the importance of sexual fantasies as a means of self-exploration and expression. Fantasies can serve as a bridge between our innermost desires and our lived realities. In a group setting, these fantasies can be shared and enacted, fostering intimacy and excitement among participants.

Benefits of Role-Playing in Group Scenarios

1. **Enhanced Communication:** Engaging in role-play requires clear communication about desires, boundaries, and consent. This practice can improve overall communication skills within the group, leading to more satisfying encounters.

2. **Increased Arousal:** Role-playing can heighten arousal by introducing novel elements and breaking away from routine sexual practices. The thrill of embodying a character or scenario can amplify sexual tension and excitement.

3. **Exploration of Power Dynamics:** Role-playing often involves the exploration of power dynamics, which can be particularly stimulating in group settings. Participants can negotiate roles that reflect their fantasies, whether they involve dominance, submission, or equal power dynamics.

4. **Emotional Connection:** Sharing and enacting fantasies can deepen emotional bonds among participants. The vulnerability involved in role-playing fosters trust and intimacy, enriching the overall experience.

Common Challenges

While role-playing can be highly rewarding, it is not without its challenges. Here are some potential issues to consider:

1. **Miscommunication:** Without clear communication, role-playing scenarios can lead to misunderstandings or discomfort. It is crucial to establish a safe environment where participants feel comfortable expressing their needs and boundaries.

2. **Fear of Judgment:** Participants may worry about being judged for their fantasies or the roles they wish to explore. Creating a non-judgmental atmosphere is essential for encouraging open expression.

3. **Emotional Triggers:** Some role-playing scenarios may inadvertently trigger past traumas or emotional responses. It is vital to have pre-established discussions about potential triggers and to agree on safe words or signals that allow participants to pause or stop if needed.

Practical Examples of Role-Playing Scenarios

1. **The Fantasy Encounter:** Participants can create a scenario based on a shared fantasy, such as a chance meeting in a bar where flirtation leads to a group sexual encounter. This setup allows for playful interactions, teasing, and building tension before engaging in sexual activities.

2. **Power Exchange Dynamics:** One participant may take on a dominant role, while others assume submissive roles. This dynamic can be explored through verbal commands, physical restraint, or guiding the actions of others. Clear boundaries and consent are paramount in these scenarios.

3. **Character Play:** Participants can embody characters from movies, books, or personal fantasies. For example, a group may decide to role-play as characters from a popular fantasy series, allowing for imaginative interactions that enhance the erotic experience.

4. **Themed Parties:** Organizing a themed party can provide a structured environment for role-playing. Themes such as "Masquerade Ball" or "Futuristic Fantasy" can inspire participants to dress up and create scenarios that align with the theme, adding an extra layer of excitement.

Incorporating Fantasies into Group Dynamics

To effectively incorporate fantasies into group play, consider the following strategies:

1. **Pre-Play Discussions:** Prior to the encounter, hold discussions about each participant's fantasies and comfort levels. This conversation can help identify common interests and establish boundaries.

2. **Written Agreements:** Create a written agreement outlining each participant's fantasies, boundaries, and safe words. This document can serve as a reference point to ensure everyone feels secure and respected.

3. **Trial Runs:** For those new to role-playing, consider starting with lighter scenarios or shorter role-play sessions. This approach allows participants to ease into the experience and build confidence over time.

4. **Feedback Sessions:** After the encounter, hold a feedback session to discuss what worked well and what could be improved. This practice can enhance communication and foster a culture of openness in future group encounters.

In conclusion, incorporating role-playing and fantasies into group sexual encounters can significantly enhance pleasure and connection. By understanding the theoretical underpinnings, recognizing potential challenges, and implementing practical strategies, participants can create a safe and exhilarating environment for exploration. Embrace the opportunity to ride the wave of pleasure together, unlocking new dimensions of erotic fulfillment.

Engaging in Dirty Talk and Vocalization for Heightened Pleasure

Dirty talk and vocalization are powerful tools in enhancing sexual experiences, particularly in group scenarios. Engaging in these practices can amplify arousal, foster intimacy, and create a stimulating atmosphere that encourages exploration and connection among partners. This section delves into the theory behind dirty talk, potential challenges, and practical examples to help you harness the full potential of vocal expression in group sexual encounters.

The Theory Behind Dirty Talk

Dirty talk involves using sexually charged language to express desires, fantasies, or encouragement during intimate moments. It can serve multiple functions, including:

+ **Enhancing Arousal:** Verbal expression can stimulate the mind, which is a significant component of sexual arousal. The brain's response to erotic language can trigger physiological reactions, such as increased heart rate and heightened sensitivity.

+ **Creating Intimacy:** Sharing fantasies and desires through dirty talk can foster emotional connections between partners. This vulnerability can deepen trust and enhance the overall experience.

+ **Encouraging Exploration:** Vocalizing desires can open the door for partners to explore new dimensions of pleasure, leading to a more fulfilling sexual experience.

The psychological basis for the effectiveness of dirty talk lies in its ability to tap into the erotic imagination. According to the *Dual Control Model of Sexual Response*, individuals experience sexual arousal through a complex interplay of excitatory and inhibitory processes. Engaging in dirty talk can activate the excitatory system, leading to a more intense sexual experience.

Challenges of Dirty Talk

While dirty talk can enhance pleasure, it may also present challenges, particularly in group settings. Some common issues include:

+ **Insecurity and Self-Consciousness:** Individuals may feel anxious about how their words will be received or fear judgment from others. This self-consciousness can inhibit vocal expression.

+ **Miscommunication:** Different partners may have varying comfort levels with explicit language, leading to misunderstandings or discomfort. It is crucial to establish a shared vocabulary and boundaries.

+ **Cultural and Personal Differences:** Personal backgrounds and cultural norms may influence comfort with dirty talk. Some individuals may find it empowering, while others may feel it is inappropriate.

Addressing these challenges requires open communication and a willingness to explore comfort levels with all partners involved.

Practical Examples of Dirty Talk

To effectively engage in dirty talk, consider the following strategies and examples:

+ **Compliments and Affirmations:** Expressing appreciation for a partner's body or performance can boost confidence and arousal. For example, saying, "I love the way you touch me" or "You feel amazing inside me" can heighten pleasure.

+ **Describing Actions:** Verbalizing what you or your partners are doing can create a vivid mental image. For instance, "I can feel you getting harder" or "I love the way your lips feel on my skin" can enhance the experience.

- **Expressing Desires:** Sharing what you want to do or what you enjoy can guide partners and intensify arousal. Phrases like, "I want you to take me harder" or "I can't wait to taste you" can be highly effective.

- **Fantasy Sharing:** In a group context, sharing fantasies can create a collective atmosphere of excitement. For example, saying, "Imagine us all together, exploring each other's bodies" can encourage exploration and connection.

- **Encouragement and Feedback:** Providing positive reinforcement can enhance the experience for everyone. Phrases like, "That feels so good" or "Don't stop, I want more" can motivate partners to continue their actions.

Techniques for Effective Vocalization

To maximize the impact of dirty talk, consider these techniques:

- **Tone and Volume:** Adjusting your tone and volume can add layers of meaning to your words. A whisper can create intimacy, while a louder voice can convey urgency and excitement.

- **Timing:** Timing is crucial in dirty talk. Engaging in vocalization during peak moments of arousal can amplify the experience. Pay attention to the rhythm of the encounter and speak when the energy is high.

- **Non-Verbal Cues:** Complement verbal expressions with non-verbal cues, such as eye contact, body language, and physical touch. This holistic approach can enhance the overall experience.

Conclusion

Engaging in dirty talk and vocalization during group sexual encounters can significantly enhance pleasure and intimacy. By understanding the theory behind these practices, addressing potential challenges, and employing practical techniques, you can create a stimulating and fulfilling experience for yourself and your partners. Embrace the power of your voice and let it guide you on a journey of exploration, connection, and heightened pleasure.

Understanding and Stimulating Erogenous Zones in Group Settings

Erogenous zones are areas of the body that, when stimulated, can lead to heightened sexual arousal and pleasure. Understanding these zones is crucial in group sexual encounters, where multiple partners may be involved, and the dynamics can vary significantly from one-on-one interactions.

Theoretical Background

The concept of erogenous zones is rooted in human anatomy and psychology. According to Masters and Johnson, the most sensitive areas of the body, such as the genitals, breasts, and inner thighs, are rich in nerve endings that respond to touch, pressure, and temperature changes. However, erogenous zones can extend beyond these commonly recognized areas. The brain plays a significant role in sexual arousal, and individual experiences, preferences, and psychological factors can influence what is considered pleasurable.

Common Erogenous Zones

1. **Clitoris**: Often cited as the most sensitive area for individuals with vulvas, the clitoris has more than 8,000 nerve endings and is crucial for achieving orgasm. 2. **G-Spot**: Located a few inches inside the vaginal canal on the anterior wall, stimulation of the G-spot can lead to intense pleasure and potential orgasm. 3. **Nipples**: For many, nipple stimulation can be incredibly arousing, triggering a strong sexual response. 4. **Inner Thighs**: Light caresses or kisses along the inner thighs can build anticipation and arousal. 5. **Neck and Ears**: Areas such as the neck and earlobes can be sensitive to kissing, nibbling, or whispering, enhancing intimacy and arousal. 6. **Feet and Toes**: Often overlooked, foot massages or gentle touches can be intensely pleasurable for some individuals.

Challenges in Group Settings

In a group sexual encounter, the challenge lies in the diversity of preferences and comfort levels among participants. Here are some common problems that may arise:
   - **Miscommunication**: With multiple people involved, it can be easy for someone to misinterpret cues or boundaries, leading to discomfort or disengagement. - **Overstimulation**: Some individuals may feel overwhelmed by simultaneous stimulation from multiple partners, which can detract from the experience. - **Jealousy and Competition**: The presence of multiple partners can evoke feelings of jealousy or insecurity, which may hinder the ability to relax and enjoy the experience.

Strategies for Effective Stimulation

To navigate these challenges and enhance pleasure through the stimulation of erogenous zones, consider the following strategies:

1. **Establish Clear Communication**: Before engaging in group play, have an open discussion about each participant's preferences and boundaries. Use clear language to articulate what feels good and what does not.

2. **Use a Team Approach**: In group settings, coordinate with partners to focus on different erogenous zones simultaneously. For example, one partner can stimulate the clitoris while another focuses on the G-spot, creating a more comprehensive experience.

3. **Practice Active Listening**: Pay attention to verbal and non-verbal cues from partners. Encourage feedback and adjustments to ensure everyone is comfortable and enjoying the experience.

4. **Explore Different Techniques**: Vary the type of stimulation used on erogenous zones. For instance, alternating between gentle caresses, firm pressure, and light teasing can keep the experience dynamic and engaging.

5. **Incorporate Sensual Elements**: Use props such as feathers, ice, or warm oils to enhance the stimulation of erogenous zones. Sensory play can introduce new sensations and intensify pleasure.

6. **Create a Safe Space**: Foster an environment where everyone feels safe to express their desires and boundaries. This atmosphere of trust can lead to more profound connections and heightened pleasure.

Examples of Erogenous Zone Stimulation in Groups

- **Clitoral Stimulation**: In a group setting, one partner can focus on direct clitoral stimulation using fingers or a toy, while another partner kisses and caresses the inner thighs, creating a layered experience of pleasure.

- **G-Spot Exploration**: One partner may penetrate vaginally while another stimulates the G-spot externally, using a combination of thrusting and circular motions to enhance the sensation.

- **Nipple Play**: While one partner massages the breasts, others can engage in kissing or licking the nipples, providing varied sensations that can lead to heightened arousal.

Conclusion

Understanding and stimulating erogenous zones in group settings can significantly enhance the pleasure and intimacy of the experience. By fostering open communication, establishing trust, and exploring diverse techniques, participants can navigate the complexities of group dynamics while maximizing pleasure for all involved. Embracing these practices not only enriches individual experiences but also strengthens connections within the group, paving the way for deeper intimacy and shared pleasure.

Enhancing Pleasure through Breathwork and Energy Circulation

Breathwork is a powerful yet often overlooked tool in enhancing sexual pleasure and intimacy, particularly in group sexual encounters. The practice of consciously controlling one's breath can significantly influence arousal, emotional connection, and overall sexual experience.   This section explores the theories behind breathwork, its impact on energy circulation within the body, and practical techniques to incorporate breathwork into group scenarios.

Theoretical Foundations of Breathwork

Breathwork is rooted in various traditions, including yoga, tantra, and mindfulness practices. The basic premise is that breath is a vital force that connects the mind, body, and spirit. In many spiritual philosophies, breath is considered a conduit for energy, often referred to as *prana* in yoga or *qi* in Chinese medicine. By focusing on breath, individuals can enhance their awareness of bodily sensations, heighten arousal, and facilitate deeper emotional connections.

$$E = \frac{1}{2}mv^2 \tag{21}$$

This equation, derived from classical mechanics, illustrates that energy is a function of mass and velocity. In the context of sexual pleasure, the "mass" can be thought of as the physical presence of the body, while "velocity" can represent the intensity and rhythm of breath, which can amplify sexual energy and arousal.

The Role of Breath in Sexual Arousal

Breath influences the autonomic nervous system, which governs physiological responses during sexual activity.   Deep, rhythmic breathing activates the parasympathetic nervous system, promoting relaxation and enhancing pleasure. Conversely, shallow or rapid breathing can trigger the sympathetic nervous system, often associated with anxiety or stress, which can inhibit pleasure.

Common Challenges

Many individuals may find it difficult to focus on their breath during intimate moments due to distractions or societal conditioning that associates breath with anxiety rather than pleasure. Common problems include:

- **Shallow Breathing:** Often a result of tension or anxiety, leading to reduced oxygen flow and diminished pleasure.

- **Disconnection:** Participants may feel disconnected from their bodies or partners, hindering emotional and physical intimacy.

- **Overthinking:** Worrying about performance or others' perceptions can disrupt natural breathing patterns.

Practical Techniques for Breathwork in Group Scenarios

To effectively incorporate breathwork into group sexual encounters, consider the following techniques:

1. **Synchronizing Breath with Partners** Encourage group members to synchronize their breathing patterns. This can create a sense of unity and shared energy. Participants can start by inhaling deeply together for a count of four, holding for a count of four, and exhaling for a count of six. This rhythmic breathing can enhance emotional connection and increase overall arousal.

$$\text{Breath Cycle} = \text{Inhale (4s)} + \text{Hold (4s)} + \text{Exhale (6s)} \qquad (22)$$

2. **Breath of Fire** A technique borrowed from yoga, the Breath of Fire involves rapid, rhythmic inhalations and exhalations through the nose. This invigorating breath can heighten sexual energy and excitement. To practice, participants can sit comfortably, inhale deeply, and then exhale forcefully while drawing the navel in towards the spine, repeating this for several cycles.

3. **Tantric Breathing** Incorporate tantric breathing techniques, which focus on slow, deep breaths that engage the diaphragm. Participants can visualize energy flowing through their bodies with each inhalation and exhalation. This visualization can enhance the sensation of pleasure and intimacy.

Energy Circulation Techniques

In addition to breathwork, understanding energy circulation is crucial in maximizing pleasure. Energy can be visualized as flowing through the body along pathways known as meridians or chakras. Here are some techniques to enhance energy circulation during group encounters:

1. Grounding Techniques Encourage participants to ground themselves by feeling their connection to the earth. This can be done through visualization or physical touch, such as placing hands on the ground. Grounding helps stabilize energy and enhances the ability to connect with others.

2. Circulating Energy Participants can practice circulating energy by forming a circle and passing energy through touch. One partner can initiate a gentle touch, and as it travels around the circle, everyone can focus on breathing deeply and visualizing energy flowing through their bodies.

3. Utilizing Sound and Breath Incorporate vocalizations, such as humming or moaning, synchronized with breath. This practice not only enhances personal pleasure but also creates a resonant energy within the group, fostering a deeper connection among participants.

Conclusion

Breathwork and energy circulation are powerful tools that can significantly enhance pleasure during group sexual encounters. By understanding the theoretical foundations and overcoming common challenges, participants can explore new dimensions of intimacy and connection. Incorporating these techniques into group play can lead to profound experiences of pleasure, emotional bonding, and personal growth. Embrace the power of breath to ride the waves of pleasure and connection in your next group encounter.

Incorporating Sex Toys and Props for Added Stimulation

In the context of group sexual encounters, the use of sex toys and props can significantly enhance pleasure, facilitate exploration, and create a dynamic atmosphere of shared enjoyment. By integrating these tools into your experience, you can amplify arousal, cater to diverse preferences, and foster a sense of adventure among participants.

Understanding the Role of Sex Toys and Props

Sex toys can serve various purposes, from enhancing physical pleasure to facilitating emotional connection. They can help individuals explore their bodies in new ways, stimulate erogenous zones, and provide a shared experience that enhances group dynamics. Whether you are using vibrators, dildos, or other props, it's essential to consider how these tools can be incorporated into your group play to maximize pleasure for everyone involved.

Types of Sex Toys and Their Uses

- **Vibrators:** These devices can be used on oneself or shared among partners. They can stimulate the clitoris, G-spot, or other sensitive areas, making them ideal for enhancing arousal during group encounters. Consider using a variety of vibrators, such as bullet vibrators for targeted stimulation or wand massagers for broader coverage.

- **Dildos:** These phallic-shaped toys can be used for penetration or external stimulation. They come in various sizes, shapes, and materials, allowing participants to choose based on their preferences. Incorporating dildos can create opportunities for partners to explore different sensations and configurations.

- **Anal Toys:** Anal beads, butt plugs, and prostate massagers can add a new layer of pleasure for participants interested in anal play. These toys can be used solo or during group interactions to stimulate the anus and surrounding areas, enhancing overall arousal.

- **Bondage Gear:** Incorporating props like cuffs, ropes, or blindfolds can introduce elements of BDSM into your group play. This can heighten excitement and anticipation, allowing participants to explore power dynamics and trust in a safe environment.

- **Sensory Props:** Items such as feathers, ice cubes, or hot wax can stimulate the senses and create unique sensations. Experimenting with temperature play or gentle teasing can heighten arousal and encourage participants to explore their limits.

Incorporating Toys into Group Dynamics

To effectively incorporate sex toys and props into group encounters, consider the following strategies:

1. **Establish Guidelines:** Before introducing toys, discuss preferences and boundaries with all participants. This ensures that everyone feels comfortable and safe, fostering an environment where exploration can thrive.

2. **Encourage Exploration:** Allow participants to explore the toys at their own pace. Encourage them to communicate their desires and preferences, creating an open dialogue that enhances connection and intimacy.

3. **Rotate Toys:** Consider implementing a rotation system where toys are passed around among participants. This not only allows everyone to experience the pleasure of the toys but also encourages communication about what feels good and what doesn't.

4. **Pair Toys with Techniques:** Combine the use of toys with specific techniques, such as synchronized movements or shared breathing exercises, to deepen the connection among participants. For example, using a vibrator while engaging in mutual touch can create a powerful synergy of sensations.

5. **Mindful Usage:** Encourage participants to remain mindful of their bodies and the sensations they are experiencing. This can enhance the overall experience and help individuals achieve deeper levels of pleasure.

Addressing Common Concerns

While incorporating sex toys can be exciting, it is essential to address potential concerns:

+ **Hygiene:** Ensure that all toys are cleaned before and after use. Discuss safe practices for sharing toys, such as using condoms on penetrative toys or ensuring that everyone is aware of hygiene protocols.

+ **Compatibility:** Not all toys are suitable for all participants. Discuss preferences and comfort levels to ensure that everyone is on the same page regarding the types of toys being used.

+ **Emotional Reactions:** Some individuals may feel vulnerable or insecure when using toys in a group setting. Encourage open communication and check in with participants to address any concerns or discomfort.

Examples of Group Play Scenarios with Toys

1. **Vibrator Circles:** Participants can sit in a circle and take turns using a vibrator on themselves or on a partner. This allows for exploration of different sensations and fosters a sense of community and connection.

2. **Dildo Relay:** Partners can engage in a relay-style play where they take turns using a dildo on each other, exploring different techniques and positions. This encourages communication and experimentation.

3. **Bondage and Sensory Play:** Incorporate bondage gear alongside sensory props to create a multi-layered experience. For instance, blindfolded participants can be teased with feathers while others use vibrators to stimulate them, heightening anticipation and pleasure.

4. **Group Edging:** Participants can use toys to bring each other close to orgasm without allowing release. This can be a thrilling way to build sexual tension and enhance the eventual climax.

Conclusion

Incorporating sex toys and props into group sexual encounters can open up a world of possibilities for pleasure and exploration. By communicating openly, establishing guidelines, and fostering a sense of trust, participants can create an enriching experience that maximizes pleasure for everyone involved. Embrace the boldness of exploration, and remember that the journey to pleasure is as important as the destination.

Exploring Different Sexual Activities and Configurations in Groups

Group sexual encounters offer a diverse array of sexual activities and configurations that can enhance pleasure and intimacy among participants. Understanding these configurations not only maximizes individual enjoyment but also fosters connection and communication within the group. This section delves into various sexual activities and configurations, providing theoretical insights, potential challenges, and practical examples to help you navigate these experiences with confidence and creativity.

1. Theoretical Foundations of Group Sexual Configurations

Group sexual configurations can be categorized into several types based on the number of participants and the nature of interactions. The most common configurations include threesomes, orgies, and polyamorous gatherings. Each configuration presents unique dynamics that can influence the sexual experience.

1.1 Threesomes Threesomes involve three participants engaging in sexual activities. This configuration can take various forms, such as MFM (male-female-male), FMF (female-male-female), or even same-gender combinations. The dynamics of a threesome often hinge on the relationships between the participants. For example, two partners may invite a third person to enhance their sexual experience, which can lead to feelings of excitement and novelty. However, it is essential to establish clear boundaries and communication to mitigate potential jealousy or insecurity.

1.2 Orgies An orgy typically involves multiple participants engaging in sexual activities simultaneously. This configuration allows for a variety of interactions, from one-on-one encounters to group play. The sheer number of participants can amplify the sexual energy in the room, creating an exhilarating atmosphere. However, the complexity of managing consent and boundaries increases with the number of participants, making effective communication crucial.

1.3 Polyamorous Gatherings Polyamorous gatherings focus on the emotional connections between multiple partners, often emphasizing love and intimacy alongside sexual activities. These configurations can vary widely, from casual meetups to established polycule relationships. The key to successful polyamorous encounters lies in open communication and mutual respect, ensuring that all participants feel valued and understood.

2. Common Sexual Activities in Group Settings

The activities engaged in during group sexual encounters can range from intimate to adventurous. Here are several common activities that can enhance the experience:

2.1 Group Foreplay Group foreplay serves as a critical component in building arousal and creating a sensual atmosphere. Techniques such as synchronized kissing, touching, and caressing can heighten anticipation and establish a collective rhythm. For example, participants may form a circle and take turns kissing or massaging each other, fostering intimacy and connection.

2.2 Sensory Play   Incorporating sensory play can elevate the experience by stimulating the senses in unique ways. This may involve blindfolds, feathers, or ice cubes to create contrasting sensations. Participants can take turns exploring each other's bodies while others watch, enhancing feelings of voyeurism and exhibitionism.

2.3 Role-Playing   Role-playing allows participants to explore fantasies and power dynamics within a safe environment. Whether embodying characters from popular media or creating entirely new scenarios, role-playing can add layers of excitement and creativity to the encounter. For instance, one might take on the role of a dominant figure while others play submissive roles, allowing for exploration of consent and boundaries.

3. Configurations for Enhanced Pleasure

The arrangement of bodies in a group sexual encounter can significantly impact the overall experience. Here are a few configurations that can facilitate pleasure:

3.1 The Wheel   In the wheel configuration, participants sit in a circle, facing outward, with one participant in the center. The center participant can engage with each person in the circle, creating a dynamic flow of energy and attention. This configuration allows for individual exploration while maintaining a sense of connection with the group.

3.2 The Sandwich   The sandwich configuration involves one person being "sandwiched" between two others. This setup can enhance feelings of safety and support, as the person in the middle receives attention from both sides. This arrangement can be particularly pleasurable for individuals who enjoy being the focus of attention.

3.3 The Chain   In the chain configuration, participants form a line, each engaging with the person in front and behind them. This setup encourages continuous interaction and can create a rhythmic flow of pleasure. It can also foster a sense of unity among participants, as everyone is connected in a shared experience.

4. Challenges and Considerations

While exploring different sexual activities and configurations can be exhilarating, it is essential to acknowledge potential challenges:

4.1 Communication   Effective communication is the cornerstone of any successful group sexual encounter. Participants must feel comfortable expressing their desires, boundaries, and concerns. Establishing a group agreement or safe word can facilitate open dialogue and ensure everyone is on the same page.

4.2 Jealousy and Insecurity   Feelings of jealousy or insecurity may arise during group encounters, particularly if one participant feels neglected or overshadowed. It is crucial to address these emotions openly and honestly, allowing for discussions that reinforce trust and connection.

4.3 Consent and Safety   Consent must be continuously negotiated and respected in group settings. Participants should be encouraged to check in with one another regularly, ensuring that everyone feels safe and comfortable throughout the encounter. Establishing clear guidelines around safe sex practices is also essential to protect the health and well-being of all participants.

5. Practical Examples

To illustrate these concepts, consider the following practical examples:

5.1 The Group Date   A group of friends decides to explore their sexual connections in a safe and consensual manner. They establish clear boundaries, discuss desires, and create a safe word for the evening. As they engage in group foreplay, they rotate partners, allowing everyone to experience different types of touch and intimacy.

5.2 The Themed Party   A themed party encourages participants to dress up and embody specific characters, enhancing the role-playing aspect of the encounter. Participants engage in a variety of sexual activities, from sensual massages to playful teasing, all while maintaining open communication and consent.

5.3 The Retreat   A weekend retreat focused on sexual exploration provides a safe space for individuals to connect and engage in group activities. Workshops on communication, consent, and pleasure techniques are offered, allowing participants to deepen their understanding of their desires and boundaries.

In conclusion, exploring different sexual activities and configurations in group settings can significantly enhance pleasure and intimacy. By understanding the dynamics of various configurations, engaging in diverse activities, and addressing potential challenges, participants can create fulfilling and enjoyable group sexual experiences. Remember, the key to maximizing pleasure in group scenarios lies in open communication, consent, and a willingness to explore the depths of connection and desire.

Techniques for Maintaining Arousal and Stamina in Group Encounters

Maintaining arousal and stamina during group sexual encounters is essential for maximizing pleasure and ensuring that all participants can fully engage in the experience. This section explores various techniques that can help individuals sustain their excitement and energy levels throughout the encounter.

Understanding Arousal and Stamina

Arousal and stamina are interconnected components of sexual experience. Arousal refers to the physiological and psychological state of being sexually excited, while stamina pertains to the endurance to engage in sexual activities over an extended period. The interplay between these two elements can significantly influence the quality of sexual encounters, especially in group settings.

The Role of Arousal in Group Dynamics

In group scenarios, maintaining a heightened state of arousal can facilitate deeper connections and shared pleasure among participants. Arousal can be influenced by various factors, including emotional connection, physical stimulation, and the environment. The following techniques can enhance arousal and stamina, allowing participants to ride the wave of pleasure throughout the experience.

Techniques for Maintaining Arousal

1. **Mindful Breathing:** Focusing on breath can enhance arousal by increasing oxygen flow to the body and promoting relaxation. Practicing deep, rhythmic breathing can help participants stay present in the moment, heightening sensations and emotional connections. Try the following technique:

Inhale deeply through the nose for 4 seconds, hold for 4 seconds, exhale through the

Repeat this cycle several times to enhance arousal.

2. **Sensory Stimulation:** Engage all five senses to amplify arousal. Use scented candles, soft music, or textured fabrics to create an immersive environment. Encourage participants to share what sensations excite them, leading to a more connected experience.

3. **Physical Movement:** Incorporating movement can help maintain energy levels. Participants can engage in gentle dancing, stretching, or synchronized movements to keep the body active and excited. This not only enhances stamina but also fosters a sense of unity among group members.

4. **Vocalization:** Encourage participants to express their pleasure verbally. Sounds of enjoyment can enhance arousal for both the individual and their partners. Dirty talk or simply vocalizing pleasure can create an atmosphere of excitement and connection.

5. **Edging:** This technique involves bringing oneself or a partner close to orgasm and then backing off before climaxing. Edging can prolong the sexual experience and increase the intensity of eventual orgasms. It's an excellent way to maintain arousal while building anticipation within the group.

6. **Taking Breaks:** Allowing for brief pauses can help participants regroup and recharge. During these breaks, engage in non-sexual touch, such as cuddling or massaging, to maintain intimacy and connection without the pressure of continuous sexual activity.

7. **Hydration and Nutrition:** Staying hydrated and maintaining energy levels through light snacks can prevent fatigue. Encourage participants to drink water and consider healthy snacks, such as fruits or nuts, to keep energy levels up throughout the encounter.

8. **Switching Roles and Activities:** Changing up sexual positions or activities can prevent monotony and keep arousal levels high. Encourage participants to explore different dynamics, such as switching partners or trying new techniques, to maintain excitement.

9. **Establishing a Safe Word:** Having a safe word can alleviate anxiety and enhance relaxation. When participants know they can pause or stop at any time, they can focus on pleasure rather than worry, leading to sustained arousal.

10. **Positive Affirmations:** Encourage participants to share positive affirmations about themselves and each other. Compliments can boost confidence and enhance arousal, creating a supportive and uplifting atmosphere.

Addressing Common Problems

Despite the techniques outlined, participants may encounter challenges in maintaining arousal and stamina. Here are some common issues and their solutions:

+ **Performance Anxiety:** Participants may feel pressure to perform or meet expectations. Open communication about fears and desires can alleviate anxiety and foster a supportive environment.

+ **Distractions:** External noises or interruptions can disrupt focus. Create a comfortable space, free from distractions, to help participants stay engaged in the experience.

+ **Fatigue:** Physical exhaustion can hinder stamina. Encourage regular breaks and hydration to help participants recharge and maintain energy levels.

+ **Emotional Blocks:** Past traumas or insecurities may surface during group encounters. Encourage participants to practice self-compassion and seek emotional support from partners when needed.

Conclusion

Maintaining arousal and stamina in group sexual encounters is a multifaceted endeavor that requires awareness, communication, and creativity. By employing these techniques, participants can create a dynamic and pleasurable experience that enhances intimacy and connection, ultimately leading to deeper satisfaction for all involved. Embrace the journey, and remember that pleasure is not just about the destination but the shared experience along the way.

Techniques for Multiple Orgasms in Group Scenarios

Understanding the Anatomy of the Orgasm: Clitoral, G-Spot, and Blended

Understanding the anatomy of orgasm is crucial for maximizing pleasure during group sexual encounters. Different types of orgasms—clitoral, G-spot, and blended—offer unique sensations and experiences. This section will explore each type, their physiological underpinnings, and practical implications for enhancing pleasure in group scenarios.

1. The Clitoral Orgasm

The clitoris is often regarded as the powerhouse of female pleasure. It contains approximately 8,000 nerve endings, making it one of the most sensitive areas of the human body. The clitoral network extends beyond the visible external structure, encompassing internal parts that wrap around the vaginal canal.

Physiology: The clitoral orgasm occurs primarily through direct or indirect stimulation of the clitoris. When arousal begins, blood flow increases to the clitoral area, causing it to swell and become more sensitive. This heightened sensitivity can lead to intense pleasure and, ultimately, orgasm.

Problems: Despite the clitoris's significance, many individuals may struggle to achieve clitoral orgasms due to various factors, including:

+ Lack of knowledge about their own bodies

+ Anxiety or performance pressure in group settings

+ Miscommunication with partners about preferences

Examples: In group scenarios, focusing on clitoral stimulation can be enhanced through:

+ Coordinated group foreplay, where multiple partners take turns stimulating the clitoris.

+ Utilizing sex toys, such as vibrators, that can provide consistent stimulation.

+ Engaging in techniques like oral sex, which can be particularly effective when partners work together to create a rhythm.

2. The G-Spot Orgasm

The G-spot, or Grafenberg spot, is an area located on the anterior vaginal wall, approximately 1 to 3 inches inside the vagina. When stimulated, it can lead to intense pleasure and orgasm for some individuals.

Physiology: The G-spot is thought to be an extension of the clitoral network, with many nerve endings and erectile tissue. Stimulation of the G-spot can lead to a different type of orgasm, often described as deeper and more intense than a clitoral orgasm.

Problems: Challenges associated with G-spot orgasms may include:

+ Difficulty locating the G-spot, which can vary in sensitivity among individuals.

+ Psychological barriers, such as anxiety or fear of not achieving orgasm.

+ Misinformation about the G-spot, leading to unrealistic expectations.

Examples: To facilitate G-spot orgasms in group encounters:

+ Encourage partners to explore different angles and depths of penetration to locate the G-spot.

+ Integrate hands-on techniques, where one partner stimulates the G-spot while others provide external stimulation.

+ Use of sex toys designed for G-spot stimulation can enhance the experience and make it more accessible.

3. The Blended Orgasm

A blended orgasm is a combination of clitoral and G-spot stimulation, resulting in a more holistic and intense experience. This type of orgasm can be particularly fulfilling, as it harnesses the benefits of both types.

Physiology: During a blended orgasm, the simultaneous stimulation of both the clitoris and G-spot can create a cascading wave of pleasure. This can lead to heightened arousal and a more profound sense of release.

Problems: However, achieving a blended orgasm may present its own challenges:

+ Difficulty coordinating stimulation from multiple partners.

+ Potential for overstimulation, which may lead to discomfort rather than pleasure.

+ Misalignment of partners' rhythms and techniques, causing frustration.

Examples: To achieve blended orgasms in group scenarios:

+ Establish clear communication about preferences and comfort levels.

+ Experiment with different configurations, such as a partner using their fingers for G-spot stimulation while another provides clitoral stimulation.

+ Engage in synchronized movements, where partners work together to create a rhythm that enhances pleasure for everyone involved.

Conclusion

Understanding the anatomy of orgasms—clitoral, G-spot, and blended—is essential for maximizing pleasure in group sexual encounters. By recognizing the physiological aspects and potential challenges, individuals can enhance their experiences and foster deeper connections with their partners. In the context of group play, open communication and a willingness to explore different techniques can lead to fulfilling and pleasurable experiences for all involved. Remember, every body is unique, and the journey to discovering what works best for you and your partners is part of the excitement.

$$\text{Total Pleasure} = \text{Clitoral Stimulation} + \text{G-Spot Stimulation} + \text{Emotional Connection} \tag{24}$$

Techniques for Achieving Multiple Orgasms in Women

Achieving multiple orgasms is a thrilling journey that many women can experience, characterized by a series of orgasms occurring in quick succession without a significant refractory period. Understanding the physiological and psychological aspects of female orgasm can enhance this experience, allowing for a deeper connection to one's body and pleasure.

Understanding Female Anatomy

To effectively achieve multiple orgasms, it is crucial to understand the anatomy involved:

+ **Clitoris:** The primary organ of sexual pleasure, the clitoris extends internally and is rich in nerve endings. Stimulation of the clitoris can lead to intense orgasms.

+ **G-Spot:** Located on the anterior vaginal wall, the G-spot can produce a different sensation of pleasure when stimulated. Some women report that G-spot stimulation can lead to a more profound orgasmic experience.

+ **Blended Orgasms:** Many women experience orgasms that are a combination of clitoral and G-spot stimulation, providing a richer and more varied sexual experience.

Techniques for Multiple Orgasms

1. **Build Arousal Gradually**   Gradual buildup is key to achieving multiple orgasms. Start with foreplay that focuses on stimulating the clitoris and erogenous zones. Techniques include:

+ **Gentle Touching:** Use fingers or a partner's hands to explore the body, focusing on sensitive areas like the inner thighs, breasts, and clitoris.

+ **Kissing and Caressing:** Engage in intimate kissing and caressing to heighten arousal before moving to more direct stimulation.

2. **Focus on Breathing**   Breath control can significantly enhance sexual pleasure and orgasmic potential. Techniques include:

+ **Deep Breathing:** Inhale deeply through the nose, allowing the abdomen to expand, and exhale slowly through the mouth. This practice can help maintain relaxation and increase arousal.

+ **Breath Synchronization:** If engaging with a partner, synchronize breathing to create a sense of unity and shared pleasure.

3. **Experiment with Edging**   Edging involves bringing oneself or a partner close to orgasm and then backing off before climaxing. This technique can increase the intensity of subsequent orgasms. Steps include:

+ **Identify the Edge:** Recognize the sensations that signal nearing orgasm and communicate these with your partner.

+ **Pause and Change Stimulation:** When approaching the edge, reduce stimulation or switch techniques (e.g., from clitoral to vaginal stimulation) to prolong arousal.

4. Utilize Kegel Exercises   Kegel exercises strengthen the pelvic floor muscles, which can enhance orgasmic intensity and control. To perform Kegels:

+ **Identify Muscles:** Locate the pelvic floor muscles by stopping urination midstream.

+ **Practice:** Contract these muscles for 3-5 seconds, then relax for the same duration. Repeat this for several sets throughout the day.

5. Explore Different Positions   Certain sexual positions can facilitate deeper stimulation and help achieve multiple orgasms. Consider:

+ **Missionary with Elevated Hips:** Placing a pillow under the hips can tilt the pelvis and enhance G-spot stimulation.

+ **Doggy Style:** This position allows for deep penetration and can stimulate the G-spot effectively.

6. Incorporate Vibrators and Sex Toys   Using vibrators can provide consistent stimulation that may be difficult to achieve manually. Techniques include:

+ **Clitoral Stimulation:** Use a clitoral vibrator while engaging in penetrative sex to enhance pleasure.

+ **Dual-Stimulation Toys:** Consider toys designed for both vaginal and clitoral stimulation, providing simultaneous pleasure.

7. Communicate Openly with Partners   Effective communication about desires, boundaries, and preferences is essential for a fulfilling sexual experience. Strategies include:

+ **Discuss Fantasies:** Share desires and fantasies with partners to create a comfortable environment for exploration.

+ **Provide Feedback:** Give and receive feedback during encounters to adjust techniques and enhance pleasure.

Addressing Common Challenges

While the journey to multiple orgasms can be exhilarating, there may be challenges. Common issues include:

- **Performance Anxiety:** Worrying about achieving multiple orgasms can create stress. Focus on the pleasure of the moment rather than the outcome.

- **Physical Discomfort:** If discomfort arises, communicate with partners to adjust positions or techniques.

- **Emotional Blocks:** Past traumas or emotional issues may inhibit sexual pleasure. Consider seeking support from a therapist specializing in sexual health.

Conclusion

Achieving multiple orgasms is a deeply personal and unique experience for every woman. By understanding anatomy, employing various techniques, and fostering open communication, women can explore their sexual potential and embrace the joy of multiple orgasms. Remember, the journey is as important as the destination; savor each moment and celebrate your body's capacity for pleasure.

Techniques for Achieving Multiple Orgasms in Men

Achieving multiple orgasms is often seen as a mystical experience reserved for women, yet men can also tap into this potential through a combination of physical techniques, mental strategies, and emotional readiness. Understanding the physiological processes involved in male orgasm and ejaculation is crucial for those seeking to experience multiple climaxes.

Understanding Male Anatomy and Orgasm

To appreciate how to achieve multiple orgasms, it's essential to understand male anatomy and the orgasmic process. The male orgasm typically involves a series of physiological changes, including increased heart rate, heightened blood flow to the genitals, and muscle contractions in the pelvic region.

The male orgasm can be broken down into two phases:

1. **Emission Phase**: This is when sperm is propelled into the urethra, preparing for ejaculation. 2. **Ejaculation Phase**: This is the expulsion of semen from the body, often accompanied by intense pleasure.

After ejaculation, men usually experience a refractory period—a recovery time during which it is challenging to achieve another erection or orgasm. However, with practice and the right techniques, some men can learn to bypass this refractory period, allowing for multiple orgasms.

Techniques for Achieving Multiple Orgasms

1. Edging   Edging, or the practice of bringing oneself close to orgasm and then stopping before ejaculation, can help men learn to control their arousal levels. This technique allows for heightened sensitivity and prolonged pleasure, which can lead to multiple orgasms.
   How to Edge:

+ Begin with stimulating activities that you find pleasurable.

+ As you approach the point of orgasm, slow down or stop stimulation.

+ Focus on your breathing and allow arousal to subside slightly before resuming stimulation.

+ Repeat this process several times before allowing yourself to climax.

2. Kegel Exercises   Kegel exercises strengthen the pelvic floor muscles, which play a critical role in orgasm control. By enhancing these muscles, men can increase their ability to experience multiple orgasms.
   How to Perform Kegel Exercises:

+ Identify the right muscles by stopping urination midstream.

+ Once identified, contract these muscles for 3-5 seconds, then relax for the same duration.

+ Aim for 10-15 repetitions, three times a day.

3.   Mindfulness and Breath Control   Mindfulness practices can significantly enhance sexual experiences, including the ability to achieve multiple orgasms. By focusing on the sensations in the body and maintaining a calm, centered state, men can better navigate their arousal levels.
   Breath Control Technique:

+ Inhale deeply through the nose, filling your abdomen with air.

+ Hold the breath for a count of four.

+ Exhale slowly through the mouth, focusing on relaxing your body.

+ Use this technique during sexual activity to maintain control over arousal.

4. **Tantric Practices** Tantric sex emphasizes connection, energy flow, and prolonged pleasure. Incorporating Tantric practices can help men explore their orgasmic potential more fully.
   Basic Tantric Technique:

+ Engage in slow, deliberate movements that focus on intimacy and connection with your partner.

+ Synchronize your breathing with your partner's to enhance energy exchange.

+ Explore different forms of touch and stimulation to increase arousal without rushing toward climax.

5. **Exploring Different Types of Stimulation** Experimenting with various forms of stimulation can lead to multiple orgasms. This can include:
   - **Prostate Stimulation**: Often referred to as the "male G-spot," stimulating the prostate can lead to intense orgasms. Use fingers or toys designed for prostate stimulation while maintaining other forms of stimulation.
   - **Sensory Play**: Incorporating elements such as feathers, ice, or heat can heighten arousal and lead to heightened orgasmic experiences.

Common Challenges

While the potential for multiple orgasms is exciting, there are common challenges that men may face:

1. **Refractory Period** The refractory period can vary significantly among individuals. Patience and practice are key; some men may find that their refractory period shortens over time with consistent practice of the techniques outlined.

2. **Performance Anxiety** Worrying about performance can hinder the ability to relax and enjoy the experience. Focusing on pleasure rather than performance can help alleviate anxiety.

3. Communication with Partners   Open dialogue with partners about desires and boundaries is essential. Ensuring both partners are comfortable and engaged can enhance the experience and facilitate multiple orgasms.

Conclusion

Achieving multiple orgasms as a man is not only possible but can also be a deeply fulfilling experience. By employing techniques such as edging, Kegel exercises, mindfulness, Tantric practices, and exploring various forms of stimulation, men can unlock their potential for multiple climaxes. Emphasizing communication, patience, and self-exploration will further enhance this journey into pleasure, allowing for a richer and more satisfying sexual experience.

Techniques for Achieving Multiple Orgasms in Non-Binary Individuals

Achieving multiple orgasms is a journey of exploration and understanding, particularly for non-binary individuals who may experience arousal and orgasm in unique and diverse ways. This section will delve into the techniques that can enhance sexual pleasure and facilitate the experience of multiple orgasms, while also addressing the specific physiological and psychological considerations relevant to non-binary bodies.

Understanding Non-Binary Sexuality

Non-binary individuals may possess a variety of sexual anatomies and experiences that can influence their orgasmic potential. It is crucial to recognize that the path to orgasm is not universal; rather, it is shaped by personal preferences, anatomical variations, and individual emotional landscapes. The following techniques aim to honor this diversity and empower non-binary individuals in their pursuit of pleasure.

1. Emphasizing Self-Exploration

Self-exploration is foundational for understanding one's own body and sexual responses. Non-binary individuals should feel encouraged to engage in solo pleasure practices that allow them to discover their unique erogenous zones and preferences. Techniques such as:

+ **Mirror Exploration:** Using a mirror to view one's body can enhance body awareness and acceptance. This technique allows for the visualization of different sensations and responses during self-exploration.

+ **Mindful Masturbation:** Focusing on the sensations rather than the goal of orgasm can lead to a more profound understanding of what feels good. This practice encourages non-binary individuals to explore various rhythms, pressures, and areas of stimulation.

2. Utilizing the Power of Breath

Breathwork is a powerful tool for enhancing arousal and facilitating multiple orgasms. Techniques include:

+ **Deep Breathing:** Engaging in deep, rhythmic breathing can help relax the body and increase blood flow to the genitals, enhancing sensitivity and arousal.

+ **Breath Control:** Practicing breath control during stimulation can help manage arousal levels. For example, inhaling deeply during stimulation and exhaling slowly can create a rhythm that prolongs pleasure and delays climax, paving the way for multiple orgasms.

3. Exploring Different Stimulation Techniques

Non-binary individuals can benefit from experimenting with various forms of stimulation that resonate with their bodies. Techniques include:

+ **Clitoral Stimulation:** For those with external genitalia, focusing on the clitoris—using fingers, toys, or external stimulation—can lead to heightened arousal. The clitoris has over 8,000 nerve endings, making it a prime target for pleasure.

+ **G-Spot and Prostate Stimulation:** For individuals with internal anatomy, exploring the G-spot or prostate can unlock new pathways to orgasm. Techniques such as gentle pressure and rhythmic movements can be employed to stimulate these areas effectively.

+ **Combination Techniques:** Engaging in simultaneous stimulation of both the clitoris and G-spot/prostate can amplify sensations and increase the likelihood of experiencing multiple orgasms. Communication with partners about what feels good is essential in these scenarios.

4. Edging and Prolonged Arousal

Edging, or the practice of bringing oneself close to orgasm and then backing off, is an effective technique for building sexual tension. This practice can lead to more intense orgasms and increase the chances of experiencing multiple orgasms. The process involves:

- **Identifying the Point of No Return:** Learning to recognize the sensations that indicate approaching orgasm allows for better control over the orgasmic response.

- **Delaying Orgasm:** Once at the edge, non-binary individuals can switch techniques or take a break to prolong arousal, experimenting with different forms of stimulation or even changing positions.

5. Incorporating Tantric Practices

Tantric practices can enhance sexual experiences by promoting connection, mindfulness, and prolonged pleasure. Non-binary individuals may find value in:

- **Sensual Breathing:** Synchronizing breath with a partner can deepen the emotional connection and enhance physical sensations.

- **Energy Circulation:** Visualizing and circulating sexual energy throughout the body can amplify arousal and lead to multiple orgasmic experiences.

6. Communication and Feedback

Effective communication is vital in any sexual encounter, especially in group settings. Non-binary individuals should feel empowered to express their desires, boundaries, and feedback openly. Techniques include:

- **Verbal Affirmations:** Encouraging partners to share what feels good can enhance the experience for everyone involved.

- **Non-Verbal Cues:** Developing a system of non-verbal signals can help communicate pleasure levels and desires without interrupting the flow of the encounter.

7. Aftercare and Emotional Support

Aftercare is crucial for emotional well-being after sexual encounters. Non-binary individuals should prioritize:

+ **Physical Comfort:** Engaging in cuddling, gentle touch, or simply resting together can foster a sense of safety and connection.

+ **Emotional Check-Ins:** Discussing feelings and experiences post-encounter can help process emotions and strengthen bonds with partners.

Conclusion

The journey to achieving multiple orgasms as a non-binary individual is deeply personal and multifaceted. By embracing self-exploration, utilizing breathwork, experimenting with various stimulation techniques, and prioritizing communication and aftercare, non-binary individuals can unlock their orgasmic potential. Remember, pleasure is not a destination but an ever-evolving exploration, and every experience is an opportunity for growth and joy.

Exploring Extended Orgasm and Edging in Group Play

Extended orgasm and edging are powerful techniques that can enhance pleasure and intimacy during group sexual encounters. These practices not only amplify the physical sensations experienced by participants but also foster emotional connections and shared experiences. This section delves into the theory behind extended orgasm and edging, addresses potential challenges, and provides practical examples to help you navigate these techniques in group scenarios.

Theoretical Framework

Extended orgasm refers to the ability to prolong the orgasmic experience, allowing for multiple peaks of pleasure without a full release. This phenomenon is rooted in the understanding of the sexual response cycle, which includes the phases of excitement, plateau, orgasm, and resolution. By manipulating these phases, individuals can experience heightened arousal and a series of orgasms that may last longer than traditional experiences.

Edging, or orgasm denial, involves bringing oneself or a partner to the brink of orgasm and then stopping stimulation before reaching climax. This practice can create a build-up of sexual tension, leading to more intense orgasms when release is finally allowed. According to research by [?], the anticipation and delay associated with edging can significantly enhance sexual satisfaction.

Challenges and Considerations

While exploring extended orgasm and edging in group settings can be exhilarating, there are several challenges to consider:

+ **Communication:** Clear communication is essential to ensure that all participants are comfortable with the pace and intensity of stimulation. Establishing safe words or signals can help manage the experience.

+ **Physical Limits:** Participants should be aware of their own bodies and limits. Overstimulation can lead to discomfort or pain, which may detract from the experience. It's important to check in with one another regularly.

+ **Emotional Dynamics:** Edging can intensify emotions, including arousal and frustration. Participants should be prepared for the possibility of heightened feelings of jealousy or insecurity, especially if one partner is receiving more attention than others.

Practical Examples

To successfully incorporate extended orgasm and edging into group play, consider the following techniques:

1. **Group Edging Sessions:** Begin with a consensual agreement among all participants to engage in edging. Set a timer for a specific duration, such as 15 minutes. During this time, focus on stimulating each other without allowing anyone to reach orgasm. Use a variety of techniques, including oral, manual, and toy stimulation, while maintaining open communication about comfort levels.

2. **Breath Control and Synchronization:** Encourage participants to synchronize their breathing. This not only helps build a collective energy but also enhances the connection between partners. As everyone approaches the edge of orgasm, take deep breaths together, creating a shared rhythm that amplifies the tension.

3. Varying Stimulation Techniques: Experiment with different types of stimulation, such as alternating between gentle teasing and more intense pleasure. This variation can help participants stay engaged and excited while avoiding climax. For example, one partner may use a vibrator on another while others provide sensual touch or engage in kissing.

4. Gradual Release: After a period of edging, allow one participant to climax while the others continue to stimulate them. This can create a visually stimulating experience for the group, as well as a sense of collective pleasure. Following this, allow others to take turns, ensuring that everyone has an opportunity to experience both the build-up and release.

5. Incorporating Tantric Practices: Tantric techniques can enhance the experience of extended orgasm and edging. Focus on energy exchange through eye contact, synchronized movements, and mindful touch. Encourage participants to explore their sensations and emotions, fostering a deeper connection that transcends physical pleasure.

Conclusion

Exploring extended orgasm and edging in group play can be a transformative experience that deepens intimacy and enhances pleasure. By understanding the theoretical underpinnings, addressing potential challenges, and utilizing practical techniques, participants can create a fulfilling and empowering sexual environment. Remember, the key to success lies in communication, consent, and a willingness to explore together.

Utilizing Kegel Exercises and Pelvic Floor Muscles for Orgasm Control

Kegel exercises, named after Dr. Arnold Kegel who developed them in the 1940s, are a powerful tool for enhancing sexual pleasure and achieving orgasm control. These exercises target the pelvic floor muscles, which support the bladder, uterus, and rectum. Strengthening these muscles can lead to improved sexual function, increased orgasm intensity, and better control over the timing of orgasm.

Understanding the Pelvic Floor Muscles

The pelvic floor is a group of muscles that form a supportive hammock at the base of the pelvis. These muscles are responsible for several critical functions, including:

+ Supporting pelvic organs (bladder, uterus, rectum)

+ Controlling urination and bowel movements

+ Enhancing sexual pleasure and orgasmic potential

To locate these muscles, try stopping urination midstream; the muscles you engage to do this are your pelvic floor muscles.

The Benefits of Kegel Exercises

The regular practice of Kegel exercises can yield several benefits:

+ **Increased Orgasm Intensity:** Strengthened pelvic floor muscles can lead to stronger contractions during orgasm, enhancing pleasure.

+ **Improved Orgasm Control:** By learning to contract and relax these muscles, individuals can gain better control over the timing and intensity of their orgasms.

+ **Enhanced Sexual Experience:** A strong pelvic floor can improve overall sexual function and satisfaction, making sexual encounters more pleasurable.

+ **Support for Sexual Health:** Kegel exercises can help in recovery from childbirth, improve bladder control, and reduce the risk of pelvic organ prolapse.

How to Perform Kegel Exercises

To perform Kegel exercises effectively, follow these steps:

1. **Identify the Right Muscles:** As mentioned, locate your pelvic floor muscles by stopping urination midstream.

2. **Get Comfortable:** You can perform Kegel exercises while lying down, sitting, or standing. Choose a position that feels comfortable for you.

3. **Contract the Muscles:** Tighten your pelvic floor muscles and hold the contraction for 3 to 5 seconds. Imagine trying to lift the pelvic floor upwards.

4. **Relax:** Release the contraction and relax the muscles for an equal amount of time.

5. **Repeat:** Aim for 10 to 15 repetitions, three times a day.

Integrating Kegel Exercises into Sexual Practice

To maximize the benefits of Kegel exercises during sexual encounters, consider the following strategies:

* **Focus on Breathing:** Incorporate deep, rhythmic breathing while performing Kegel exercises. This can enhance relaxation and increase arousal.

* **Combine with Other Techniques:** Use Kegel contractions in conjunction with other arousal techniques, such as clitoral stimulation or erotic massage, to amplify pleasure.

* **Practice Edging:** While engaging in sexual activity, practice contracting your pelvic floor muscles just before the point of orgasm. This can help delay ejaculation and build arousal.

* **Experiment with Timing:** Try contracting during penetration or while receiving oral sex to explore how it enhances sensations for you and your partner.

Common Problems and Solutions

While Kegel exercises are generally safe, some individuals may encounter challenges:

* **Difficulty Identifying Muscles:** If you're struggling to locate your pelvic floor muscles, consider consulting a pelvic floor therapist for guidance.

* **Overexertion:** Avoid overdoing the exercises, as this can lead to muscle fatigue or discomfort. Gradually increase the intensity and duration of your contractions.

* **Inconsistent Practice:** Like any muscle group, the pelvic floor requires regular exercise for optimal results. Set reminders or incorporate Kegels into your daily routine.

Conclusion

Utilizing Kegel exercises and strengthening the pelvic floor muscles can significantly enhance sexual experiences and provide greater control over orgasms. By incorporating these exercises into your sexual wellness routine, you can unlock new levels of pleasure and intimacy, making group encounters even more fulfilling. Remember, the journey to sexual empowerment is personal and unique; embrace the process and enjoy the ride!

Incorporating Tantric Practices for Prolonged Pleasure

Tantra is an ancient spiritual practice that emphasizes the connection between the body, mind, and spirit. When applied to sexual encounters, particularly in group scenarios, Tantric practices can enhance pleasure, intimacy, and connection among participants. By focusing on breath, energy, and presence, individuals can experience prolonged pleasure and multiple orgasms in a supportive and consensual environment.

Theoretical Foundations of Tantra

At its core, Tantra teaches that sexual energy is a powerful force that can be harnessed for personal growth and spiritual enlightenment. Key concepts in Tantric philosophy include:

+ **Kundalini Energy:** This is the primal energy believed to reside at the base of the spine. Through Tantric practices, individuals aim to awaken this energy, allowing it to rise through the chakras, leading to heightened states of awareness and pleasure.

+ **Chakras:** These are energy centers within the body that correspond to different physical, emotional, and spiritual aspects of the self. Engaging with these centers can enhance sexual experiences and facilitate emotional release.

+ **Presence and Mindfulness:** Tantric practices emphasize being fully present in the moment, which can deepen the connection between partners and enhance the overall experience of pleasure.

Common Tantric Techniques for Prolonged Pleasure

Incorporating Tantric practices into group sexual encounters can be transformative. Here are some techniques that can be employed:

1. Breathwork:

    + Synchronizing breath with partners can create a shared rhythm, enhancing connection and arousal.

    + Techniques such as *ujjayi breath* (victorious breath) can amplify sensations and prolong pleasure. To practice, inhale deeply through the nose, constricting the throat slightly to create a soft sound, and exhale slowly through the mouth.

2. **Eye Gazing:**

   + Engaging in prolonged eye contact can foster intimacy and trust among partners.   This practice encourages vulnerability and connection, heightening arousal.

   + Set a timer for 3-5 minutes of uninterrupted eye contact, allowing participants to explore the energy flowing between them.

3. **Slow and Sensual Touch:**

   + Encourage participants to explore each other's bodies slowly, focusing on sensitive areas and varying pressure and speed. This can build anticipation and prolong pleasure.

   + Use a feather, silk, or other soft materials to stimulate the skin gently, enhancing sensory awareness.

4. **Energy Exchange:**

   + Participants can practice passing energy through touch, breath, or movement. This can create a sense of unity and shared pleasure in the group.

   + Form a circle and pass energy by touching hands or connecting through breath, visualizing energy flowing between participants.

5. **Extended Orgasm Techniques:**

   + Teach participants to recognize the signs of approaching orgasm and to use techniques such as *edging*—the practice of bringing oneself close to orgasm and then backing off—to prolong pleasure.

   + Encourage participants to communicate their sensations and desires, creating a feedback loop that enhances the experience for everyone involved.

Addressing Common Challenges

While incorporating Tantric practices can be rewarding, participants may encounter challenges, including:

+ **Discomfort with Vulnerability:** Some individuals may struggle with being vulnerable in a group setting. Establishing a safe and consensual environment is crucial. Encourage open communication about feelings and boundaries.

+ **Difficulty in Staying Present:** The mind may wander during practice. Encourage participants to gently bring their focus back to their breath, sensations, and the connection with their partners.

+ **Managing Expectations:** Participants may have preconceived notions about what Tantric practices should achieve. Emphasize that the goal is not necessarily to reach orgasm but to explore pleasure and connection.

Examples of Tantric Practices in Group Scenarios

Here are some practical examples to illustrate how Tantric practices can be incorporated into group sexual encounters:

+ **Tantric Circle:** Participants sit in a circle, taking turns to share their desires and intentions. Each person can then engage in a brief session of eye gazing or breath synchronization with their chosen partner, fostering intimacy and trust.

+ **Partnered Breathwork:** In pairs, participants can practice synchronized breathing while gently touching each other. As they breathe together, they can explore different types of touch, allowing energy to flow and build arousal.

+ **Guided Sensual Massage:** One partner can guide another in a sensual massage, focusing on slow, deliberate movements while maintaining eye contact and breath synchronization. This can create a deeply intimate experience and enhance overall pleasure.

Incorporating Tantric practices into group sexual encounters can lead to profound experiences of pleasure and connection. By focusing on breath, energy, and presence, participants can explore new dimensions of intimacy, ultimately enhancing their sexual experiences and fostering a deeper sense of community and trust.

Techniques for Non-Gendered Individuals in Group Scenarios

In the vibrant tapestry of human sexuality, non-gendered individuals bring unique perspectives and experiences to group sexual encounters. Recognizing and honoring this diversity is essential for creating an inclusive and pleasurable environment. In this section, we will explore techniques tailored to non-gendered individuals, focusing on enhancing pleasure, fostering connection, and ensuring comfort in group scenarios.

Understanding Non-Gendered Experiences

Non-gendered individuals may identify outside the binary constructs of male and female, encompassing a range of identities such as genderqueer, agender, and genderfluid. Understanding the nuances of these identities can significantly impact the dynamics of group sexual encounters. It is crucial to approach each individual with openness and respect, acknowledging their unique preferences and boundaries.

Communication as a Foundation

Effective communication is the cornerstone of any successful sexual encounter, particularly in group settings. Non-gendered individuals may face specific challenges related to their identities, such as misgendering or assumptions about their sexual roles. To mitigate these issues:

- **Establish Clear Communication:** Encourage all participants to share their pronouns and preferred terms. This practice fosters an inclusive atmosphere and minimizes discomfort.

- **Set Boundaries:** Non-gendered individuals should feel empowered to articulate their boundaries and desires. Encourage open dialogue about what feels good and what does not.

- **Utilize Check-Ins:** Regularly check in with each participant during the encounter. Simple questions like, "How are you feeling?" or "Is this working for you?" can enhance comfort and connection.

Exploring Techniques for Pleasure

When it comes to pleasure, non-gendered individuals may have diverse anatomical and psychological responses. Here are some techniques that can enhance their experience in group scenarios:

1. **Sensory Exploration**   Encourage non-gendered individuals to explore their bodies and sensations without the constraints of traditional gender roles. This exploration can include:

- **Sensory Deprivation:** Using blindfolds or noise-canceling headphones can heighten other senses, allowing individuals to focus on touch, taste, and smell.

+ **Temperature Play:** Experimenting with hot and cold sensations, such as ice cubes or warm oils, can create new and exciting experiences.

2. **Inclusive Positioning**   Group dynamics can be enhanced by incorporating sexual positions that allow for equal participation and pleasure among all individuals, regardless of gender identity. Consider:

+ **Circles and Clusters:** Arranging participants in a circle or cluster can promote intimacy and facilitate easier access to one another's bodies.

+ **Fluid Positions:** Encourage fluidity in positions, allowing individuals to shift and change roles as desired, thus avoiding rigid expectations based on gender.

3. **Emphasizing Non-Genital Touch**   Non-genital touch can be particularly empowering for non-gendered individuals. Techniques may include:

+ **Full-Body Massage:** Encourage partners to explore each other's bodies through massage, focusing on erogenous zones beyond the genitals, such as the neck, back, and inner thighs.

+ **Kissing and Caressing:** Emphasize the importance of kissing and caressing as forms of connection that can be deeply pleasurable without being explicitly sexual.

Navigating Emotional Dynamics

Emotional dynamics in group settings can be complex, especially for non-gendered individuals who may feel marginalized. Addressing these dynamics involves:

+ **Creating Safe Spaces:** Establish an environment where all participants feel safe to express their emotions and vulnerabilities. This can be achieved through group agreements and aftercare practices.

+ **Compassionate Listening:** Encourage participants to practice active listening, validating each other's feelings and experiences without judgment.

Aftercare and Emotional Support

Aftercare is essential for all individuals, particularly for non-gendered participants who may experience unique emotional responses. Consider the following practices:

+ **Individualized Aftercare:** Tailor aftercare to the needs of non-gendered individuals, which may include cuddling, verbal reassurance, or quiet time to process the experience.

+ **Group Reflection:** Engage in a group reflection session post-encounter, allowing participants to share their feelings, insights, and any concerns they may have.

Conclusion

Incorporating techniques tailored for non-gendered individuals in group sexual encounters not only enhances pleasure but also fosters a sense of belonging and acceptance. By prioritizing communication, exploring diverse techniques, and providing emotional support, we can create enriching experiences that honor the full spectrum of human sexuality. Embrace the beauty of diversity and ride the wave of pleasure together, celebrating the unique contributions of every participant.

Enhancing Orgasms through Mental Stimulation and Mindfulness

In the realm of sexual pleasure, the mind is a powerful ally. The connection between mental stimulation, mindfulness, and orgasmic experiences is profound, influencing not only the intensity of pleasure but also the ability to achieve multiple orgasms. This section delves into the theoretical underpinnings of this relationship, the common challenges individuals face, and practical strategies to enhance orgasms through mental engagement and mindfulness.

Theoretical Framework

The connection between mental stimulation and orgasm can be understood through various psychological and physiological theories. The *Dual Control Model* of sexual response posits that sexual arousal is governed by both excitatory and inhibitory processes in the brain. This model highlights that mental stimulation can serve as a significant excitatory factor, enhancing sexual arousal and orgasm potential.

Moreover, the concept of *mindfulness*—defined as maintaining a moment-by-moment awareness of our thoughts, feelings, bodily sensations, and surrounding environment—plays a crucial role in sexual experiences. Mindfulness encourages individuals to focus on the present moment, reducing distractions and enhancing sensory experiences. Research shows that mindfulness can lead to increased sexual satisfaction and a greater ability to achieve orgasm, particularly in group settings where external stimuli may be overwhelming.

Common Challenges

Despite the potential benefits of mental stimulation and mindfulness, many individuals encounter challenges that can hinder their ability to fully engage in these practices. Common issues include:

+ **Distraction:** In group settings, the presence of multiple partners can lead to sensory overload, making it difficult to focus on one's own pleasure or that of others.

+ **Performance Anxiety:** Concerns about how one is perceived by others can create mental barriers that inhibit relaxation and pleasure.

+ **Negative Self-Talk:** Internal dialogues that criticize one's body or sexual performance can detract from the enjoyment of the moment.

+ **Emotional Blocks:** Past traumas or unresolved emotional issues may surface during intimate encounters, causing distraction and discomfort.

Strategies for Enhancement

To harness the power of mental stimulation and mindfulness, individuals can adopt several strategies that promote a more fulfilling sexual experience:

1. Mindful Breathing Techniques Engaging in mindful breathing can ground individuals in the present moment and enhance arousal. Practicing deep, rhythmic breathing can help calm the nervous system and increase blood flow to erogenous zones. For example, try the following technique:

1. Inhale deeply through the nose for a count of four, allowing the abdomen to expand.

2. Hold the breath for a count of four.

3. Exhale slowly through the mouth for a count of six, feeling the body relax with each breath.

Repeat this cycle several times, focusing on the sensations in the body and the rhythm of the breath.

2. Visualization Techniques   Visualization can be a powerful tool for enhancing arousal and orgasm. Imagining erotic scenarios or recalling pleasurable experiences can stimulate the mind and body. For instance, individuals might visualize:

+ A fantasy involving their partners, focusing on the details of touch, sound, and sensation.

+ A previous intimate encounter that brought them immense pleasure, recalling the feelings and sensations experienced.

Encouraging partners to share their fantasies can also heighten arousal and create a shared mental space that fosters connection.

3. Sensory Awareness Exercises   Focusing on sensory experiences can enhance mindfulness during sexual encounters. Individuals can practice tuning into their senses by:

+ Paying attention to the texture of skin, the warmth of breath, and the sounds of pleasure.

+ Engaging in sensory play with partners, using blindfolds or restraints to heighten awareness of touch.

+ Experimenting with different sensory stimuli, such as temperature play with ice or warm oils, to enhance the erotic experience.

4. Affirmations and Positive Self-Talk   Replacing negative self-talk with positive affirmations can shift one's mindset and enhance the sexual experience. Before engaging in group play, individuals can practice affirmations such as:

"I am deserving of pleasure,"
"My body is beautiful and capable of experiencing joy,"
"I trust my partners and embrace this experience."

Repeating these affirmations can help cultivate a positive mindset, reducing anxiety and enhancing enjoyment.

5. Engaging in Group Dynamics Mindfully   In group settings, it is crucial to maintain open lines of communication and check in with partners regularly. Practicing mindfulness during these interactions can foster a sense of safety and connection. Techniques include:

- Establishing safe words and signals to ensure everyone feels comfortable expressing their needs and boundaries.

- Taking moments to pause and breathe together, cultivating a shared sense of presence.

- Encouraging verbal and non-verbal feedback during encounters to enhance mutual understanding and pleasure.

Conclusion

Enhancing orgasms through mental stimulation and mindfulness is an empowering journey that can lead to profound pleasure and connection in group sexual encounters. By understanding the interplay between mind and body, addressing common challenges, and implementing practical strategies, individuals can unlock new dimensions of pleasure. Embracing mindfulness not only enriches the sexual experience but also fosters deeper emotional connections with partners, ultimately leading to more fulfilling and joyful group dynamics.

In the pursuit of pleasure, remember: the mind is not just a spectator; it is an essential participant in the symphony of sexual ecstasy.

Techniques for Post-Orgasmic Bliss and Recovery in Group Sexual Encounters

In the realm of group sexual encounters, the experience does not conclude with the climax; rather, it transitions into a crucial phase of post-orgasmic bliss and recovery. This period is essential for emotional bonding, physical recovery, and the overall enhancement of sexual experiences. Understanding how to navigate this stage can deepen connections and ensure that all participants feel valued and cared for.

Understanding Post-Orgasmic States

After orgasm, individuals often enter a state of relaxation and euphoria, influenced by the release of hormones such as oxytocin and prolactin. These hormones foster feelings of intimacy and satisfaction, but they can also lead to vulnerability. It's essential to acknowledge that the post-orgasmic phase can vary widely among individuals, influenced by emotional states, personal experiences, and the dynamics of the group.

Techniques for Enhancing Post-Orgasmic Bliss

1. **Mindful Breathing:** After an intense sexual experience, participants can engage in mindful breathing exercises. This practice helps to ground individuals, allowing them to reconnect with their bodies and emotions. Inhale deeply for a count of four, hold for four, and exhale for six. Repeat this cycle several times to promote relaxation and emotional clarity.

2. **Sensual Touch and Cuddling:** Physical touch post-orgasm can reinforce bonds and create a sense of safety. Encourage participants to engage in gentle caresses, cuddling, or holding hands. This non-sexual intimacy can significantly enhance feelings of connection and comfort. Research indicates that skin-to-skin contact releases oxytocin, further deepening emotional ties.

3. **Verbal Affirmations:** Open communication about the experience is vital. Encourage participants to share their feelings, express gratitude, and provide positive feedback. Simple affirmations like "I enjoyed that" or "You were amazing" can enhance feelings of acceptance and validation, fostering a supportive environment.

4. **Hydration and Nutrition:** Post-play, it's essential to replenish the body. Encourage participants to hydrate with water or electrolyte-rich beverages. Light snacks such as fruits or nuts can help restore energy levels and maintain blood sugar balance, promoting overall well-being.

5. **Gentle Movement or Stretching:** Engaging in gentle stretches or light movement can help release any residual tension in the body. This practice not only aids physical recovery but also encourages participants to reconnect with their bodies in a loving and nurturing way.

Addressing Potential Challenges

While the post-orgasmic phase can be blissful, it may also present challenges such as emotional vulnerability, fatigue, or feelings of insecurity. Here are some strategies to navigate these potential issues:

- **Emotional Check-Ins:** Encourage participants to check in with themselves and each other about their emotional states. This practice can help identify any feelings of discomfort or insecurity, allowing for open dialogue and support.

- **Recognizing Individual Needs:** Each person may have different needs during recovery. Some may prefer solitude, while others might seek connection. Respecting these preferences is crucial for maintaining a positive group dynamic.

- **Aftercare Agreements:** Prior to engaging in group encounters, establishing aftercare agreements can provide clarity and comfort. Discussing what each participant needs after play—whether it's cuddling, space, or conversation—can help set expectations and reduce anxiety.

The Importance of Aftercare in Group Dynamics

Aftercare is not just a personal practice; it's a collective responsibility. In group scenarios, ensuring that everyone feels cared for and supported is paramount. Here are some key points to consider:

- **Inclusivity in Aftercare:** Make it a group norm to check in with everyone after the encounter. This practice fosters a sense of community and shared responsibility, ensuring that no one feels isolated or overlooked.

- **Creating a Safe Space:** Establish a safe and comfortable environment for post-play discussions. This space should feel inviting and non-judgmental, allowing participants to express themselves freely.

- **Encouraging Reflection:** Aftercare can also involve reflecting on the experience as a group. Discuss what worked, what didn't, and how everyone felt. This reflection can enhance future encounters and promote personal growth.

Conclusion

Navigating the post-orgasmic phase in group sexual encounters is an opportunity for deepening connections and fostering emotional intimacy. By implementing mindful practices, addressing challenges, and prioritizing aftercare, participants can enhance their overall experience, ensuring that pleasure extends beyond the climax. Remember, the journey of pleasure is as important as the destination, and every moment of connection contributes to a richer, more fulfilling sexual experience.

Beyond the Orgasm: Emotional Connection and Aftercare in Group Play

Emotional Intimacy and Connection in Group Settings

Cultivating Emotional Connection with Group Partners

Cultivating emotional connections within group sexual encounters is a multifaceted process that requires intentionality, openness, and vulnerability. Emotional intimacy can enhance the overall experience, fostering deeper bonds and shared pleasure among participants. Here, we explore various strategies and theories that can facilitate emotional connection in group settings, alongside potential challenges and practical examples.

Understanding Emotional Connection

Emotional connection can be defined as a deep sense of understanding and mutual regard between individuals. In the context of group sexual encounters, this connection can be nurtured through shared experiences, effective communication, and an environment of trust and safety. Theories such as *Attachment Theory* suggest that our early relationships shape how we connect with others. Understanding your attachment style—be it secure, anxious, or avoidant—can provide insights into how you engage with partners in group settings.

Creating a Safe Environment

To cultivate emotional connections, it is crucial to establish a safe environment where participants feel comfortable expressing their feelings and desires. This can be achieved by:

- **Setting Ground Rules:** Establishing clear guidelines about consent, boundaries, and communication can help create a sense of safety. For instance, participants might agree to use a safe word or signal to pause or stop the encounter if anyone feels uncomfortable.

- **Encouraging Open Dialogue:** Open communication fosters trust. Encourage participants to share their thoughts, feelings, and concerns before, during, and after the encounter. This can include discussing what each person is looking for in the experience and any past experiences that might influence their comfort levels.

- **Practicing Active Listening:** Engaging in active listening—where participants fully concentrate, understand, respond, and remember what is being said—can deepen emotional bonds. For example, during discussions, reflect back what you hear and ask clarifying questions to show you value your partner's input.

Advantages and Challenges of Emotional Intimacy in Group Scenarios

Emotional intimacy in group sexual encounters can be a double-edged sword, offering both enriching experiences and potential pitfalls. Understanding these dynamics is crucial for navigating the complexities of pleasure and connection in group settings.

Advantages of Emotional Intimacy

Enhanced Connection   Emotional intimacy fosters a sense of connection that can deepen the pleasure experienced by all participants. When individuals feel emotionally safe and connected, they are more likely to express their desires and boundaries openly, leading to a more satisfying experience. This connection can be likened to the concept of *secure attachment*, where individuals feel safe to explore their sexuality without fear of judgment or rejection [?].

Increased Trust   Trust is foundational in any intimate encounter, and in group scenarios, it becomes even more critical. Emotional intimacy helps to build trust among participants, allowing them to feel secure in their interactions. This trust can enhance the overall experience, as individuals are more willing to explore their boundaries and engage in new activities when they feel supported by their partners [1].

Shared Vulnerability Group encounters often involve a level of vulnerability that can be both exhilarating and daunting. When participants share their vulnerabilities, it can create a powerful bond that enhances emotional intimacy. This shared experience can lead to feelings of compersion, where individuals find joy in each other's pleasure, thus enriching the group dynamic [?].

Collective Pleasure Emotional intimacy can amplify the pleasure experienced in group settings. When individuals are emotionally connected, they often synchronize their arousal and pleasure, creating a collective energy that can lead to heightened experiences of ecstasy. This phenomenon can be explained through the lens of *social facilitation theory*, which posits that the presence of others can enhance performance and pleasure in social contexts [?].

Challenges of Emotional Intimacy

Jealousy and Insecurity While emotional intimacy can foster connection, it can also evoke feelings of jealousy and insecurity. Participants may struggle with the fear of being replaced or not being enough, which can lead to tension within the group. Addressing these feelings openly is essential to prevent them from undermining the experience. Effective communication strategies, such as *nonviolent communication* (NVC), can help participants express their feelings without blame or criticism [?].

Emotional Overload Group scenarios can sometimes lead to emotional overload, particularly for individuals who are highly sensitive or empathetic. The intensity of shared experiences can be overwhelming, leading to emotional fatigue or withdrawal. It is crucial for participants to recognize their limits and take breaks as needed, practicing self-care techniques to manage emotional energy effectively [?].

Differing Levels of Intimacy In a group setting, participants may have varying levels of emotional intimacy with each other, which can create imbalance and discomfort. Some may desire deeper connections, while others may prefer a more casual interaction. This disparity can lead to misunderstandings and hurt feelings. Establishing clear communication about individual needs and desires before engaging in group play can help mitigate these challenges [?].

Navigating Group Dynamics   The dynamics of a group can shift rapidly, and emotional intimacy can complicate these changes. For instance, if one participant develops a closer bond with another, it may inadvertently create a rift within the group.   Participants must be vigilant about maintaining open lines of communication and addressing any shifts in dynamics promptly to ensure that everyone feels included and valued.

Conclusion

Emotional intimacy in group sexual encounters can significantly enhance the experience, fostering connection, trust, and collective pleasure.   However, it also presents challenges such as jealousy, emotional overload, and the need to navigate complex group dynamics.   By prioritizing open communication, establishing boundaries, and practicing self-care, participants can harness the advantages of emotional intimacy while mitigating its challenges, leading to a more fulfilling and pleasurable group experience.

Nurturing Emotional Bonds and Establishing Trust

Nurturing emotional bonds and establishing trust within group sexual encounters is paramount to ensuring a fulfilling and pleasurable experience for all participants. Emotional intimacy enhances the overall quality of the encounter, making it not only about physical pleasure but also about connection and mutual respect.

The Importance of Emotional Bonds

Emotional bonds are the invisible threads that connect individuals, creating a sense of safety and belonging.   In group sexual encounters, these bonds can significantly impact the dynamics of the experience.   When participants feel emotionally connected, they are more likely to communicate openly, express their desires and boundaries, and engage in a more profound exploration of pleasure.   Research in psychology suggests that strong emotional bonds can lead to increased satisfaction in sexual relationships (Mikulincer & Shaver, 2007).

Establishing Trust: The Foundation of Group Dynamics

Trust is the cornerstone of any intimate relationship, and its importance is magnified in group settings. Establishing trust involves several key components:

+ **Vulnerability:** Participants must feel safe to express their desires, fears, and boundaries without fear of judgment. Vulnerability fosters openness, which is essential for deep emotional connections.

+ **Consistency:** Trust is built over time through consistent behavior. When partners demonstrate reliability in their actions and words, it reinforces the sense of safety within the group.

+ **Transparency:** Open communication about intentions, desires, and boundaries helps to create an environment of honesty. This transparency allows participants to navigate their feelings and expectations effectively.

Practical Strategies for Nurturing Emotional Bonds

To nurture emotional bonds and establish trust in group sexual encounters, consider the following strategies:

1. Open Communication Encourage open dialogues before, during, and after encounters. This can include discussing fantasies, boundaries, and any concerns participants may have. For example, a pre-play meeting can help everyone articulate their desires and limits, setting a positive tone for the experience.

2. Group Check-Ins Implement regular check-ins during the encounter. This can be as simple as asking, "How is everyone feeling?" or "Is there anything anyone wants to adjust?" These check-ins promote emotional awareness and allow participants to voice their needs in real time.

3. Shared Experiences Engage in activities that foster connection outside of sexual play. This can include group outings, shared meals, or even just casual conversations. Building a rapport outside the bedroom can enhance emotional bonds and create a more relaxed atmosphere during encounters.

4. Aftercare Rituals Aftercare is crucial in nurturing emotional bonds. Taking time after the encounter to reconnect, share feelings, and provide physical comfort can strengthen the emotional ties among participants. This may involve cuddling, discussing the experience, or simply enjoying each other's company in a relaxed setting.

Addressing Challenges in Emotional Bonding

While nurturing emotional bonds is essential, challenges may arise. Here are some common issues and strategies to address them:

1. **Jealousy and Insecurity** Jealousy can undermine trust and emotional connections. To combat this, encourage open discussions about feelings of jealousy. Acknowledge these emotions without judgment and explore the root causes together. This process can foster understanding and empathy among group members.

2. **Miscommunication** Miscommunication can lead to misunderstandings and hurt feelings. To minimize this risk, emphasize the importance of active listening. Encourage participants to paraphrase what they hear to ensure clarity. For example, "What I hear you saying is..." can help confirm understanding.

3. **Emotional Overwhelm** In some cases, the intensity of group encounters can lead to emotional overwhelm. It is vital to create an environment where participants feel comfortable expressing when they need a break or want to step back. Establishing a safe word or signal can facilitate this process.

Examples of Nurturing Emotional Bonds

Consider the following scenarios that illustrate the importance of nurturing emotional bonds:

+ **Scenario 1: The Pre-Play Meeting** - A group of friends decides to engage in a sexual encounter together. Beforehand, they hold a meeting where each person shares their boundaries, desires, and any past experiences that might impact the encounter. This open dialogue creates a foundation of trust and understanding.

+ **Scenario 2: Post-Encounter Reflection** - After a group play session, participants gather to discuss their feelings about the experience. They share what they enjoyed, any discomforts they felt, and how they can improve future encounters. This reflection helps reinforce emotional connections and allows for growth.

Conclusion

Nurturing emotional bonds and establishing trust in group sexual encounters is essential for creating a safe, pleasurable, and fulfilling experience. By prioritizing open communication, shared experiences, and aftercare, participants can foster deeper connections that enhance their sexual encounters. Addressing challenges such as jealousy and miscommunication with empathy and understanding further solidifies these bonds, ensuring that everyone involved feels valued and respected. Ultimately, these emotional connections not only enrich the group experience but also contribute to personal growth and exploration in the realm of sexuality.

Bibliography

[1] Mikulincer, M., & Shaver, P. R. (2007). *Attachment in Adulthood: Structure, Dynamics, and Change*. Guilford Press.

Building Emotional Resilience and Coping Mechanisms in Group Play

Group sexual encounters can be exhilarating, but they can also stir up a whirlwind of emotions. Building emotional resilience is crucial for navigating the complexities of these experiences. Emotional resilience refers to the ability to adapt to stress and adversity, allowing individuals to bounce back from challenging situations. In the context of group play, this resilience can help participants manage feelings of jealousy, insecurity, and anxiety, ultimately enhancing the overall experience.

Understanding Emotional Resilience

Emotional resilience is not an innate trait; it can be cultivated over time through conscious effort and practice. According to Dr. Susan Kobasa's research on stress and resilience, three key components contribute to emotional resilience:

- **Commitment:** Engaging fully in experiences and relationships.

- **Control:** Believing in one's ability to influence outcomes.

- **Challenge:** Viewing difficulties as opportunities for growth.

In group sexual encounters, these components can manifest in various ways. For instance, commitment to open communication can foster trust among participants, while a sense of control can empower individuals to express their needs and boundaries. Viewing emotional challenges as opportunities for personal growth can enhance the overall experience and deepen connections with others.

Common Emotional Challenges in Group Play

1. **Jealousy:** It's natural to feel jealous in a group setting, especially when multiple partners are involved. Jealousy can stem from insecurities about one's desirability or fear of losing a partner's attention.

2. **Insecurity:** Participants may feel inadequate compared to others, leading to anxiety about performance or acceptance within the group.

3. **Overwhelm:** The intensity of multiple interactions can be emotionally overwhelming, causing individuals to feel lost or disconnected.

4. **Fear of Judgment:** Concerns about how others perceive one's body, desires, or sexual performance can create barriers to enjoyment.

Coping Mechanisms for Emotional Resilience

To navigate these emotional challenges, participants can develop effective coping mechanisms:

1. **Open Communication** Establishing a culture of open communication is paramount. Participants should feel safe expressing their feelings, desires, and concerns. Regular check-ins before, during, and after encounters can help address any issues that arise and foster a supportive environment.

2. **Setting Boundaries** Clearly defined boundaries can alleviate feelings of insecurity and jealousy. Each participant should articulate their limits and preferences, ensuring that everyone's comfort levels are respected.

3. **Mindfulness Practices** Mindfulness techniques, such as deep breathing or grounding exercises, can help individuals stay present and manage overwhelming emotions. For example, a simple breathing exercise can be practiced before entering a group scenario to center oneself:

$$\text{Inhale for 4 seconds} \quad \text{Hold for 4 seconds} \quad \text{Exhale for 4 seconds} \qquad (25)$$

This practice can reduce anxiety and promote a sense of calm.

4. **Self-Reflection** Encouraging self-reflection can help participants identify triggers and emotional responses. Journaling about experiences can provide insights into feelings of jealousy or insecurity, allowing individuals to process these emotions constructively.

5. Seeking Support Building a support network among group partners can foster emotional resilience. Participants can offer each other encouragement and understanding, creating a sense of community that enhances the experience.

Examples of Resilience in Action

Consider a scenario where an individual feels jealous during a group encounter. By practicing open communication, they express their feelings to their partners, who respond with reassurance and validation. This dialogue not only alleviates the individual's anxiety but also strengthens the emotional bonds within the group.

Another example involves an individual who feels overwhelmed by the intensity of the experience. By utilizing mindfulness techniques, they take a moment to breathe and ground themselves, allowing them to reconnect with their body and sensations. This practice enables them to fully engage in the moment rather than becoming lost in their thoughts.

Conclusion

Building emotional resilience in group sexual encounters is essential for maximizing pleasure and connection. By understanding the emotional challenges, developing coping mechanisms, and fostering open communication, participants can create a supportive environment that enhances their experiences. Emotional resilience not only enriches individual journeys but also strengthens the collective experience, leading to deeper intimacy and enjoyment in group play.

Exploring Polyamory and Relationship Configurations in Group Scenarios

Polyamory, the practice of engaging in multiple consensual romantic or sexual relationships, can significantly enhance the dynamics of group sexual encounters. Understanding various relationship configurations within polyamory allows participants to navigate their desires, boundaries, and emotional connections more effectively. This section explores the theoretical foundations of polyamory, the potential challenges it presents, and practical examples of how to incorporate these concepts into group scenarios.

Theoretical Foundations of Polyamory

Polyamory is rooted in the principles of consensual non-monogamy, where individuals have the freedom to form multiple intimate relationships. This framework challenges traditional notions of exclusivity and encourages open communication about desires and boundaries. The following theories underpin polyamorous relationships:

+ **Attachment Theory:** This psychological framework posits that the bonds we form in early life influence our relationships. In polyamorous contexts, individuals may exhibit secure, anxious, or avoidant attachment styles, which can affect how they connect with multiple partners. Understanding these styles can help individuals navigate their emotional responses and foster healthier connections within group dynamics.

+ **Communication Theory:** Effective communication is paramount in polyamorous relationships. The use of clear, honest dialogue about needs, desires, and boundaries can prevent misunderstandings and promote a supportive environment. Techniques such as nonviolent communication (NVC) can facilitate discussions about sensitive topics, enhancing emotional intimacy and trust among partners.

+ **Relational Dialectics Theory:** This theory emphasizes the tensions inherent in relationships, such as autonomy versus connection. In polyamorous settings, individuals may struggle with balancing their need for independence with their desire for intimacy. Recognizing these dialectical tensions can help partners negotiate their needs more effectively, leading to a more harmonious group experience.

Challenges in Polyamorous Group Scenarios

While polyamory can enrich group sexual encounters, it also presents unique challenges that participants must navigate:

+ **Jealousy and Insecurity:** Jealousy is a common emotion in polyamorous relationships, often stemming from fears of inadequacy or abandonment. In group scenarios, these feelings can be amplified, particularly if one partner appears to receive more attention or affection. Addressing jealousy openly and constructively is essential for maintaining group harmony.

+ **Time Management:** Balancing multiple relationships requires careful time management. Participants must navigate their schedules to ensure that all partners feel valued and prioritized. This challenge can be particularly pronounced in group settings, where the dynamics may shift as new relationships form.

+ **Emotional Labor:** Engaging in multiple relationships often involves significant emotional labor, including managing one's feelings and supporting others' emotional needs. In group scenarios, the emotional workload can increase, making it crucial for participants to practice self-care and establish boundaries to prevent burnout.

Practical Examples of Polyamory in Group Scenarios

To illustrate how polyamory can manifest in group sexual encounters, consider the following examples:

+ **Triads and Quads:** A triad consists of three individuals who are all romantically involved with one another, while a quad includes four individuals. In a group sexual encounter involving a triad, each member may prioritize their emotional connections while exploring physical intimacy together. Establishing clear communication about desires and boundaries can enhance the experience for all involved.

+ **Open Relationships:** In an open relationship, one or more partners engage in sexual encounters outside their primary relationship. For instance, a couple may invite a third partner into their sexual experiences while maintaining their emotional bond. This configuration allows for exploration and variety while prioritizing the existing relationship's health.

+ **Polyfidelity:** This arrangement involves a closed group of people who agree to be sexually and romantically exclusive with one another. In a polyfidelitous group, all members engage in group sex while maintaining emotional connections. This setup can foster a strong sense of community and trust, as participants navigate their desires together.

Conclusion

Exploring polyamory and various relationship configurations can significantly enhance the experience of group sexual encounters. By understanding the theoretical foundations of polyamory, recognizing potential challenges, and implementing practical strategies, participants can create a more fulfilling and pleasurable environment. Embracing the complexities of multiple relationships empowers individuals to connect more deeply, fostering a sense of intimacy and trust that enriches their sexual experiences.

In summary, polyamory offers a vibrant framework for exploring group dynamics, allowing individuals to ride the waves of pleasure and connection. By prioritizing communication, consent, and emotional well-being, participants can navigate the exhilarating world of group sexual encounters with confidence and joy.

Balancing Emotional Needs and Personal Autonomy in Group Encounters

In the realm of group sexual encounters, balancing emotional needs with personal autonomy is a nuanced dance that can significantly impact the overall experience for all participants. This section delves into the delicate interplay between individual desires and the collective dynamics that characterize group play.

Understanding Emotional Needs

Emotional needs in group sexual encounters can vary widely among individuals. They may include:

- **Connection:** The desire to feel emotionally connected to others, fostering a sense of belonging and intimacy.

- **Validation:** Seeking affirmation of one's worth and desirability from partners.

- **Security:** The need for reassurance regarding one's place within the group and the dynamics at play.

- **Communication:** The necessity for open dialogue about feelings, boundaries, and experiences.

Understanding these needs is crucial for creating a supportive environment. Emotional awareness can help participants articulate their feelings and expectations, paving the way for a more fulfilling experience.

The Importance of Personal Autonomy

Personal autonomy refers to the capacity to make informed, uncoerced decisions about one's own body and emotional state. In group scenarios, maintaining autonomy is vital for several reasons:

- **Empowerment:** Autonomy fosters a sense of control and empowerment, allowing individuals to engage in activities that align with their desires.

+ **Safety:** When individuals feel free to express their limits, they are more likely to engage in safe practices, both physically and emotionally.

+ **Authenticity:** Upholding personal autonomy encourages authenticity, enabling individuals to express their true selves without fear of judgment.

Challenges in Balancing Needs and Autonomy

While the importance of balancing emotional needs and personal autonomy is clear, several challenges can complicate this balance:

+ **Group Dynamics:** In group settings, the collective energy can sometimes overshadow individual needs. For instance, one person may feel pressured to participate in an activity they are uncomfortable with due to the enthusiasm of others.

+ **Jealousy and Competition:** Emotional responses such as jealousy can arise, leading to feelings of insecurity that may compromise personal autonomy. For example, witnessing a partner engage intimately with another may trigger feelings of inadequacy.

+ **Communication Barriers:** Open communication is essential, yet it can be challenging to navigate in a group. Participants may struggle to voice their needs or concerns, fearing it may disrupt the flow of the encounter.

Strategies for Balancing Emotional Needs and Autonomy

To effectively balance emotional needs and personal autonomy in group encounters, consider the following strategies:

1. **Establish Clear Communication Channels** Create an environment where open communication is encouraged. This can involve setting aside time before the encounter to discuss individual needs and boundaries. Utilizing tools such as safe words or signals can also facilitate ongoing dialogue during the encounter.

2. **Foster Emotional Awareness** Encourage participants to reflect on their emotional needs and articulate them clearly. This can be achieved through pre-play discussions or even journaling exercises that help individuals identify what they seek from the experience.

3. Emphasize Consent and Negotiation   Prioritize consent as an ongoing process rather than a one-time agreement. Encourage participants to check in with each other regularly and negotiate boundaries as the encounter unfolds. This practice reinforces both autonomy and emotional safety.

4. Create a Supportive Atmosphere   Cultivate an environment that values emotional support and understanding. This can involve affirming each other's feelings and offering reassurance, which can help mitigate feelings of jealousy or insecurity.

5. Encourage Self-Advocacy   Empower individuals to advocate for their needs and desires. This can be supported through role-playing scenarios or discussions about how to express discomfort or desire without fear of backlash.

Case Study: Navigating Emotional Needs in a Group Setting

Consider a scenario where a group of four individuals engages in a sexual encounter. One participant, Alex, feels a strong desire for emotional connection but is hesitant to express this need. As the encounter progresses, Alex observes another participant, Jamie, receiving attention from the others, leading to feelings of jealousy and insecurity.

To address this, the group had previously established a communication protocol where participants could express their feelings without judgment. Alex took a moment to voice their discomfort, stating, "I'm feeling a bit left out and would love to connect more with everyone." The group responded positively, allowing Alex to engage in a more intimate exchange with Jamie, ultimately enhancing the experience for all involved.

Conclusion

Balancing emotional needs and personal autonomy in group encounters is an ongoing process that requires mindfulness, communication, and mutual respect. By fostering an environment that values both individual desires and collective dynamics, participants can create a more enriching and pleasurable experience. Embracing this balance not only enhances personal satisfaction but also strengthens the connections forged within the group, paving the way for deeper intimacy and exploration in future encounters.

Processing Emotions and Jealousy After Group Sexual Encounters

Group sexual encounters can be exhilarating, liberating, and deeply pleasurable experiences. However, they can also elicit complex emotions, including jealousy and insecurity, which may arise during or after the encounter. Understanding how to process these emotions is crucial for maintaining healthy relationships and ensuring that all participants feel valued and respected.

Understanding Jealousy in Group Settings

Jealousy is a natural human emotion that can surface in various contexts, particularly in intimate relationships. In group sexual encounters, feelings of jealousy may arise for several reasons:

- **Comparison:** Participants may compare their desirability or performance to others in the group, leading to feelings of inadequacy.

- **Fear of Loss:** The presence of multiple partners can trigger fears of losing emotional or sexual connection with a primary partner.

- **Insecurity:** Personal insecurities about one's body, sexual abilities, or attractiveness can exacerbate feelings of jealousy.

Theoretical Framework: Attachment Theory

To better understand the emotional responses in group sexual encounters, we can draw on attachment theory, which posits that individuals form emotional bonds based on their early relationships with caregivers. These attachment styles—secure, anxious, and avoidant—can influence how individuals respond to jealousy and intimacy in group settings.

$$J = f(A, C, E) \tag{26}$$

Where:

- J = Level of Jealousy

- A = Attachment Style (Secure, Anxious, Avoidant)

- C = Communication Quality with Partners

- E = Emotional Awareness and Regulation Skills

This equation suggests that jealousy levels can be influenced by an individual's attachment style, the quality of communication with partners, and their emotional awareness and regulation skills.

Strategies for Processing Emotions and Jealousy

1. **Self-Reflection:** After a group encounter, take time to reflect on your feelings. Ask yourself questions such as:

- What specifically triggered my feelings of jealousy?

- Were these feelings rooted in insecurity or fear?

- How did my attachment style influence my emotional response?

2. **Open Communication:** Discuss your feelings with your partners. Effective communication can help to alleviate misunderstandings and reinforce trust. Use "I" statements to express your feelings without blaming others, such as:

"I felt a bit insecure when I saw you interacting closely with someone else."

3. **Reassurance and Affirmation:** Seek reassurance from your partners. Affirmations can help mitigate feelings of jealousy. A simple acknowledgment of your worth and the value of your relationship can be grounding.

4. **Mindfulness and Emotional Regulation:** Practice mindfulness techniques to help you stay present with your emotions. Techniques such as deep breathing, meditation, or grounding exercises can help you manage overwhelming feelings of jealousy.

5. **Journaling:** Writing down your thoughts and feelings can provide clarity. Reflect on what you enjoyed about the experience and what emotions surfaced. Journaling can also help you track patterns in your emotional responses over time.

Examples of Processing Emotions

Consider the following scenarios:

- **Scenario 1:** After a group encounter, Alex feels jealous when they notice their partner, Jamie, sharing an intimate moment with another participant. Instead of bottling up their feelings, Alex takes a moment to reflect on their insecurities and then discusses their feelings with Jamie, who reassures Alex of their commitment.

✦ **Scenario 2:** During a group play session, Taylor experiences jealousy when they perceive that another participant is receiving more attention. After the encounter, Taylor practices mindfulness to process their feelings and later discusses their experience with the group, fostering a supportive environment for everyone to share their emotions.

Conclusion

Processing emotions and jealousy after group sexual encounters is an essential aspect of maintaining healthy relationships and enhancing personal growth. By understanding the roots of jealousy, utilizing effective communication strategies, and practicing emotional regulation, participants can navigate their feelings and foster deeper connections with their partners. Remember, it's not only about the physical pleasure; the emotional journey is equally significant in creating fulfilling and enriching sexual experiences.

Exploring Compersion and Honoring Individual Love Languages in Groups

In the context of group sexual encounters, the concept of **compersion** emerges as a powerful emotional state that can enhance the experience for all involved. Compersion, often described as the opposite of jealousy, refers to the feeling of joy one experiences when witnessing a partner's pleasure, especially in non-monogamous or group settings. Embracing compersion can foster a deeper sense of connection, trust, and intimacy among participants, allowing everyone to ride the waves of pleasure together.

Understanding Compersion

The term *compersion* is rooted in polyamorous communities and signifies a profound emotional response. It is essential to distinguish compersion from simple happiness or satisfaction; it involves an active engagement with the feelings of others, leading to a shared emotional experience. When participants in a group scenario can feel joy for each other's pleasure, it creates a supportive atmosphere that encourages exploration and enhances overall enjoyment.

Theoretical Framework

From a psychological perspective, compersion can be understood through the lens of **empathy** and **emotional intelligence**. Empathy allows individuals to connect with the emotions of others, while emotional intelligence enables them to navigate their feelings and reactions effectively.   According to the *Theory of Mind*, individuals can attribute mental states to others, which is crucial for experiencing compersion. This ability to understand and appreciate another's emotional state can be cultivated through practice and mindfulness.

Challenges to Experiencing Compersion

Despite its benefits, many individuals struggle with feelings of jealousy and insecurity in group settings. These feelings can arise from various sources, including:

- **Insecurity about one's desirability:** Participants may fear that they will not be as attractive or desirable as others in the group.

- **Fear of abandonment:** Concerns that a partner may develop stronger feelings for someone else can lead to jealousy.

- **Societal conditioning:** Traditional views on relationships often emphasize exclusivity, making it challenging to embrace non-monogamous experiences.

To combat these challenges, it is essential to engage in open communication and self-reflection. Participants should explore their feelings, identify triggers, and work on building self-esteem and confidence.

Honoring Individual Love Languages

In addition to cultivating compersion, recognizing and honoring individual love languages can significantly enhance the emotional dynamics within a group. The concept of **love languages**, developed by Dr. Gary Chapman, identifies five primary ways people express and receive love:

- **Words of Affirmation:** Verbal expressions of affection, appreciation, and encouragement.

- **Acts of Service:** Actions taken to support and help others.

- **Receiving Gifts:** Thoughtful gestures and tangible tokens of affection.

- **Quality Time:** Dedicated time spent together, fostering connection and intimacy.

+ **Physical Touch:** Affectionate physical contact, such as hugging, kissing, and caressing.

Understanding each participant's love language can facilitate deeper connections and enhance the overall experience. For instance, if one partner thrives on words of affirmation, expressing admiration for their pleasure during a group encounter can amplify their enjoyment and foster feelings of compersion.

Practical Strategies for Cultivating Compersion and Honoring Love Languages

To integrate compersion and love languages into group sexual encounters, consider the following strategies:

1. **Open Dialogue:** Before engaging in group play, have discussions about desires, boundaries, and love languages. This sets the stage for mutual understanding and respect.

2. **Practice Mindfulness:** Encourage participants to be present and aware of their emotions and the emotions of others. This can help in recognizing feelings of joy for a partner's pleasure.

3. **Celebrate Each Other's Pleasure:** Create rituals or practices that allow participants to express joy for one another's experiences, such as verbal affirmations or cheers during intimate moments.

4. **Tailor Experiences:** Design group activities that honor individual love languages, ensuring that everyone feels valued and appreciated. For example, incorporate moments of physical touch, shared affirmations, or acts of service.

5. **Aftercare Conversations:** After the encounter, engage in discussions that reinforce feelings of connection and joy. This can include sharing what brought pleasure to each participant and expressing gratitude for each other's contributions.

Conclusion

Exploring compersion and honoring individual love languages in group sexual encounters can lead to profound emotional connections and heightened pleasure. By fostering an environment of support, understanding, and open communication, participants can navigate their feelings and embrace the joy of shared experiences. Ultimately, cultivating compersion not only enhances individual pleasure but also strengthens the bonds within the group, creating a vibrant and fulfilling sexual landscape.

Addressing Emotional Safety and Support in Group Dynamics

In the context of group sexual encounters, emotional safety is paramount. It refers to the assurance that all participants can express their feelings, desires, and boundaries without fear of judgment, rejection, or emotional harm. Establishing emotional safety not only enhances the pleasure of the experience but also fosters deeper connections among participants.

Understanding Emotional Safety

Emotional safety can be understood through the lens of attachment theory, which posits that individuals have varying attachment styles that influence their interactions and relationships. Secure attachment fosters trust and open communication, while anxious or avoidant attachment styles may lead to misunderstandings and discomfort in group settings.

$$E = \frac{C}{D} \tag{27}$$

Where:

+ E represents emotional safety,

+ C is the level of communication,

+ D is the degree of discomfort among participants.

This equation illustrates that as communication increases, emotional safety improves, thereby reducing discomfort.

Common Emotional Challenges in Group Dynamics

1. **Jealousy and Insecurity**: In group scenarios, feelings of jealousy can arise, particularly if one partner seems to receive more attention or affection. It is essential to address these feelings openly, as they can create rifts among participants.

2. **Fear of Rejection**: Participants may worry about being judged for their desires or performance. This fear can inhibit full engagement and enjoyment.

3. **Miscommunication**: With multiple participants, the potential for misunderstandings increases. Clear, ongoing communication is vital to ensure everyone feels heard and respected.

4. **Emotional Overwhelm**: The intensity of group encounters can lead to emotional overload. Participants may experience heightened feelings, and without proper support, these emotions can become overwhelming.

Strategies for Fostering Emotional Safety

1. **Establish Clear Communication Protocols**: Before engaging in group play, establish guidelines for communication. This might include regular check-ins during the encounter and a designated time for discussing feelings afterward.

2. **Use Safe Words**: Implementing safe words allows participants to express discomfort or the need for a pause without fear of disrupting the experience.

3. **Practice Active Listening**: Encourage participants to practice active listening, where they fully engage with what others are saying without planning their response while the other person is speaking. This fosters a supportive environment.

4. **Create a Pre-Play Agreement**: A pre-play agreement can outline boundaries, desires, and emotional needs. This document serves as a reference point and helps participants feel secure in their choices.

5. **Encourage Vulnerability**: Normalize sharing feelings and vulnerabilities within the group. This can be facilitated through guided discussions or check-ins where each participant shares their current emotional state.

6. **Post-Encounter Debriefing**: After the encounter, hold a debriefing session where participants can express their feelings about the experience. This can help in processing emotions and addressing any lingering concerns.

Examples of Emotional Support in Group Dynamics

- **Scenario 1**: During a group encounter, one participant feels overwhelmed and uses a safe word. The group pauses, checks in with them, and reassures them that it's okay to take a break. This action reinforces emotional safety and shows that everyone's comfort is a priority.

- **Scenario 2**: After a group play session, participants gather to discuss what they enjoyed and what could be improved. One participant expresses feelings of jealousy they experienced during the encounter. By sharing this, they open the floor for others to express similar feelings, fostering a supportive environment where everyone can learn and grow.

Conclusion

Addressing emotional safety and support in group dynamics is essential for creating a fulfilling and pleasurable experience. By implementing clear communication strategies, establishing trust, and fostering an environment of vulnerability, participants can navigate the complexities of group sexual encounters with confidence and joy. Emotional safety not only enriches the experience but also enhances the connections formed among participants, allowing for deeper intimacy and exploration of desires.

Practicing Emotional Aftercare in Group Sexual Encounters

Emotional aftercare is a crucial component of any group sexual encounter, providing a necessary space for participants to process their experiences, reinforce connections, and ensure emotional well-being. Unlike physical aftercare, which often focuses on the body's recovery, emotional aftercare addresses the psychological impacts of shared intimacy, vulnerability, and the dynamics that arise in group settings. This section will explore the importance of emotional aftercare, common challenges faced, and practical strategies for implementing effective aftercare practices.

The Importance of Emotional Aftercare

In group sexual encounters, the emotional landscape can be complex. Participants may experience a range of feelings, including joy, excitement, anxiety, jealousy, or even regret. Emotional aftercare serves several vital purposes:

- **Validation of Feelings:** Engaging in open discussions about feelings helps validate individual experiences and emotions. It allows participants to express their thoughts and feelings without fear of judgment.

- **Reinforcement of Connections:** Aftercare provides an opportunity to strengthen emotional bonds among participants. Sharing the experience can foster intimacy and enhance trust, which is essential for future encounters.

- **Processing Experiences:** Emotional aftercare allows individuals to process what occurred during the encounter, reflecting on their feelings, desires, and boundaries. This reflection can lead to personal growth and a deeper understanding of one's sexual identity.

+ **Conflict Resolution:** In group settings, misunderstandings and conflicts may arise. Aftercare provides a structured environment to address these issues, ensuring that everyone feels heard and respected.

Common Challenges in Emotional Aftercare

While emotional aftercare is essential, it is not without challenges. Participants may face difficulties such as:

+ **Vulnerability:** Sharing emotions can feel vulnerable, and some participants may struggle to articulate their feelings or fears. This can lead to emotional withdrawal or misunderstandings.

+ **Jealousy and Insecurity:** Group dynamics can exacerbate feelings of jealousy or insecurity. Participants may need additional support to navigate these emotions constructively.

+ **Diverse Emotional Responses:** Each participant may react differently to the encounter, leading to varied emotional needs. This diversity can complicate aftercare discussions and the provision of support.

+ **Time Constraints:** In some cases, participants may feel rushed to leave or may not prioritize aftercare due to social pressures. This can lead to unresolved feelings and emotional distress.

Strategies for Effective Emotional Aftercare

To ensure that emotional aftercare is both supportive and effective, consider implementing the following strategies:

1. **Create a Safe Space:** Establish a comfortable environment where participants feel safe to express their emotions. This may involve a private space where everyone can speak freely without interruptions.

2. **Encourage Open Communication:** Foster an atmosphere of open dialogue. Encourage participants to share their feelings and thoughts about the experience, using "I" statements to express personal emotions (e.g., "I felt overwhelmed when...").

3. **Practice Active Listening:** Ensure that all participants feel heard by practicing active listening. This involves not only hearing the words spoken

but also understanding the emotions behind them. Reflect back what you hear to confirm understanding.

4. **Check-In Regularly:** After the encounter, schedule regular check-ins with group members to discuss feelings and experiences. This can help participants process their emotions over time and reinforce connections.

5. **Offer Reassurance:** Acknowledge and validate any feelings of jealousy or insecurity. Reassure participants of their value and the importance of their emotional well-being. Offer affirmations that support their feelings.

6. **Engage in Physical Comfort:** Physical touch, such as cuddling or holding hands, can be incredibly soothing and help reinforce emotional bonds. However, always ensure that this is consensual and welcomed by all parties.

7. **Facilitate Group Reflection:** Encourage the group to reflect collectively on the experience. Discuss what went well, what could be improved, and how each person felt during the encounter. This can help solidify group norms and expectations for future encounters.

8. **Utilize Aftercare Rituals:** Develop specific aftercare rituals that the group can engage in post-encounter, such as sharing a meal, engaging in a group activity, or participating in a mindfulness exercise.

9. **Seek Professional Support if Needed:** If any participant struggles significantly with emotions stemming from the encounter, consider suggesting professional support, such as therapy or counseling. This can provide additional tools for processing feelings.

Conclusion

Practicing emotional aftercare in group sexual encounters is an essential aspect of fostering a supportive and healthy sexual environment. By prioritizing emotional well-being, participants can navigate the complexities of group dynamics, enhance their connections, and ensure that everyone leaves the experience feeling valued and respected. Remember, the goal of aftercare is not only to address immediate emotional needs but also to cultivate a culture of care and respect that empowers all participants in their sexual journeys.

Physical Aftercare and Self-Care Practices

Techniques for Physical Recovery and Relaxation after Group Play

Engaging in group sexual encounters can be an exhilarating experience that heightens physical pleasure and emotional connection. However, it also requires a mindful approach to recovery and relaxation afterward. This section delves into techniques that facilitate physical recovery, promote relaxation, and ensure a smooth transition back to everyday life.

Understanding the Need for Recovery

After intense physical activity, especially one involving multiple partners, the body undergoes various physiological changes. The release of hormones such as oxytocin and endorphins can lead to feelings of euphoria, but they can also be followed by fatigue and muscle tension. Recognizing the signs of physical exertion and emotional overstimulation is crucial for effective recovery. Common indicators include:

- Muscle soreness or tension

- Fatigue or lethargy

- Dehydration

- Emotional vulnerability or mood fluctuations

Addressing these symptoms through recovery techniques can enhance overall well-being and prepare individuals for future encounters.

Techniques for Recovery

1. Hydration Maintaining hydration is vital after any physical exertion. During group play, individuals often sweat and lose fluids, which can lead to dehydration. Replenishing lost fluids helps restore energy levels and supports overall bodily functions. Aim to consume water or electrolyte-rich beverages, especially those containing potassium and sodium, to aid in recovery.

$$\text{Hydration Needs} = \text{Body Weight (kg)} \times 0.033 \text{ L/kg} \qquad (28)$$

This formula provides a baseline for daily water intake, which should be adjusted based on the intensity and duration of the sexual activity.

2. Gentle Stretching and Movement   Incorporating gentle stretching exercises post-encounter can alleviate muscle tension and enhance flexibility. Stretching promotes blood circulation, which aids in the recovery of sore muscles. Focus on major muscle groups that may have been engaged during play, such as the hips, thighs, and lower back. Examples include:

- **Hip Flexor Stretch:** Kneel on one knee and push your hips forward while keeping your back straight.

- **Child's Pose:** Sit back on your heels with arms extended forward, allowing your body to relax into the stretch.

3. Sensual Massage   Engaging in a soothing massage can be an effective way to relax and recover. Not only does it relieve muscle tension, but it also fosters intimacy and connection with partners. Use warm oils or lotions to enhance the experience. Focus on areas that may feel particularly tight or sore, such as:

- Neck and shoulders

- Lower back

- Thighs and calves

Consider alternating between gentle strokes and deeper pressure to address different levels of tension.

4. Rest and Sleep   Adequate rest is crucial for recovery. Sleep allows the body to repair itself and recharge energy levels. Create a comfortable sleeping environment by:

- Using soft bedding and pillows

- Dimming lights and minimizing noise

- Practicing relaxation techniques, such as deep breathing or meditation, before sleep

Aim for 7-9 hours of quality sleep to support physical and emotional recovery.

5. Nutritional Support Post-play nutrition can significantly impact recovery. Consuming a balanced meal that includes protein, healthy fats, and carbohydrates helps replenish energy stores and repair muscle tissue. Consider meals such as:

- Grilled chicken with quinoa and vegetables
- A smoothie with spinach, banana, and protein powder
- Whole-grain toast with avocado and eggs

Emotional Recovery Techniques

Physical recovery is only one part of the post-group experience. Emotional recovery is equally important and can be facilitated through the following techniques:

1. Emotional Check-Ins After a group encounter, take time to reflect on the experience. Engage in emotional check-ins with yourself and your partners to discuss feelings, concerns, and highlights from the encounter. This practice fosters open communication and helps process any residual emotions.

2. Aftercare Rituals Engaging in aftercare rituals, such as cuddling, sharing a bath, or simply lying together in silence, can enhance feelings of safety and connection. These rituals are essential for emotional bonding and can help mitigate feelings of vulnerability that may arise after intense sexual experiences.

3. Journaling Writing about the experience can be a powerful tool for processing emotions. Consider keeping a journal where you can express thoughts, feelings, and insights about group encounters. This practice not only aids in emotional recovery but also contributes to personal growth and understanding of one's sexual journey.

Conclusion

Recovering from group sexual encounters is a multifaceted process that involves physical, emotional, and psychological components. By implementing hydration, gentle movement, sensual massage, adequate rest, and nutritional support, individuals can enhance their recovery and prepare for future experiences. Furthermore, engaging in emotional check-ins, aftercare rituals, and journaling can foster deeper connections and ensure a fulfilling journey of exploration and pleasure. Embracing these recovery techniques allows for a holistic approach to sexual well-being, empowering individuals to ride the waves of pleasure with confidence and joy.

Ensuring Safe Removal of Sex Toys and Props

In the context of group sexual encounters, the use of sex toys and props can significantly enhance pleasure, intimacy, and exploration among participants. However, ensuring their safe removal is crucial to prevent discomfort, injury, or emotional distress. This section outlines best practices, potential problems, and practical examples to guide individuals in safely removing sex toys and props after group play.

Understanding the Importance of Safe Removal

The safe removal of sex toys and props is essential for several reasons:

+ **Physical Safety:** Improper removal can lead to injuries, such as tearing, bruising, or discomfort, particularly with larger or more complex toys.

+ **Emotional Well-Being:** The end of a sexual encounter can be an emotionally charged time. Ensuring that all participants feel safe and respected during the removal process can help mitigate feelings of vulnerability or anxiety.

+ **Consent and Communication:** Clear communication about the removal process reinforces the principles of consent and mutual respect, ensuring that all parties are comfortable and aware of what to expect.

Common Problems and Challenges

While the removal of sex toys may seem straightforward, several challenges can arise:

+ **Tangled Toys:** In group scenarios, multiple toys may become tangled or intertwined, making removal more complicated.

+ **Resistance or Discomfort:** Participants may experience discomfort or resistance during the removal process, especially if they are not adequately prepared or if the toy has been in place for an extended period.

+ **Lack of Communication:** Without clear communication, misunderstandings can occur, leading to feelings of discomfort or violation of consent.

Best Practices for Safe Removal

To facilitate a safe and respectful removal process, consider the following best practices:

1. Communicate Beforehand   Before engaging in group play, discuss the use of toys and props with all participants. Establishing a clear understanding of how and when toys will be removed can alleviate anxiety and foster a sense of security. Use phrases like, "If we decide to use toys, let's agree on a signal for when it's time to remove them."

2. Use Safe Words and Signals   Implement safe words or signals that can be used during the encounter to indicate discomfort or the need to pause for removal. This ensures that all participants feel empowered to communicate their needs without fear of judgment.

3. Gradual Removal   When it comes time to remove a toy, do so gradually and gently. For example, if a toy is inserted, ensure that the individual is relaxed and ready for removal. Use a slow, steady motion, and check in with the participant: "How does that feel? Are you ready for me to take it out?"

4. Avoid Tugging or Pulling   Never yank or pull a toy out, as this can cause injury. Instead, use gentle pressure and allow the toy to come out naturally. If resistance is felt, pause and communicate with the participant to assess their comfort level.

5. Check for Discomfort   After the removal of a toy, check in with the participant to ensure they are feeling okay. Ask questions like, "How are you feeling now?" or "Do you need a moment to catch your breath?" This reinforces emotional safety and connection.

6. Clean and Care for Toys   After removal, it's essential to clean the toys properly. Discuss how to clean different materials (e.g., silicone, glass, etc.) and ensure that all participants are involved in the cleaning process, reinforcing a sense of shared responsibility.

Examples of Safe Removal Scenarios

Scenario 1: The Vibrator   In a group scenario where a vibrator is used, one partner may be holding it against another's body. As the encounter winds down, the partner controlling the vibrator should communicate: "I'm going to turn it off and gently pull it away. Is that okay?" After receiving consent, they can slowly remove the toy while maintaining eye contact and offering reassurance.

Scenario 2: The Dildo   When a dildo is used, it's crucial to ensure that the receiver is relaxed. Before removal, the user can say, "I'm going to take this out now. Let me know if you feel any discomfort." This allows the receiver to prepare mentally and physically, promoting a smoother removal process.

Scenario 3: The Restraints   If props like restraints are used, it's important to communicate clearly. For instance, one might say, "I'm going to unfasten these restraints now. Please let me know if you want me to stop at any point." This ensures a mutual understanding and respect for boundaries.

Conclusion

Ensuring the safe removal of sex toys and props in group sexual encounters is a vital aspect of fostering a positive and pleasurable experience. By prioritizing communication, consent, and emotional safety, participants can navigate the complexities of group play with confidence and care. Remember, the goal is to enhance pleasure while ensuring that all individuals feel respected and safe throughout the entire experience.

Addressing Physical Discomfort and Potential Injuries in Group Encounters

In the exhilarating realm of group sexual encounters, the potential for physical discomfort and injuries can arise, especially when multiple bodies are engaged in passionate exploration. Understanding how to recognize, address, and prevent these issues is crucial for ensuring a safe and pleasurable experience for all participants.

Understanding Common Discomforts and Injuries

Physical discomfort can manifest in various forms during group sexual activities. Common issues include:

+ **Muscle Strains:** Engaging in prolonged or unusual positions can lead to muscle fatigue or strains.

+ **Chafing:** Friction between bodies or against surfaces can cause skin irritation, especially in sensitive areas.

+ **Joint Pain:** Certain positions may place undue stress on joints, particularly in those with pre-existing conditions.

+ **Infections:** Group encounters can increase the risk of sexually transmitted infections (STIs) if safe sex practices are not adhered to.

+ **Tissue Trauma:** Rough handling or the use of toys without proper preparation can lead to tissue damage.

Recognizing the signs of discomfort early can prevent escalation into more serious injuries. Participants should be encouraged to communicate any discomfort immediately.

Preventative Measures

To minimize the risk of physical discomfort and injuries, consider the following strategies:

+ **Warm-Up:** Just as athletes warm up before engaging in physical activity, participants should engage in light stretching or gentle foreplay to prepare their bodies for movement.

+ **Position Variety:** Encourage exploration of different sexual positions that allow for comfort and ease of movement. Avoid positions that place excessive strain on any one part of the body.

+ **Lubrication:** Use adequate lubrication to minimize friction and prevent chafing. Silicone-based lubes are particularly effective for prolonged encounters.

+ **Communication:** Establish a culture of open communication where participants can express discomfort without fear. Implement a safe word or signal that can be used to pause or stop activities.

+ **Hydration and Nutrition:** Staying hydrated and maintaining energy levels through light snacks can help prevent fatigue and cramping.

Addressing Discomfort During Encounters

If discomfort arises during a group encounter, it is essential to address it promptly:

+ **Pause and Assess:** If someone expresses discomfort, pause the activity. Assess the situation collectively and determine if adjustments can be made to alleviate the issue.

‣ **Physical Adjustments:** Encourage participants to shift positions, take breaks, or change partners if necessary to redistribute physical demands.

‣ **Aftercare:** Incorporate aftercare practices that focus on physical recovery, such as gentle massage, stretching, or applying soothing lotions to irritated skin.

Case Example: Navigating Discomfort

Consider a scenario where a participant experiences discomfort due to a prolonged position that strains their back. The group can implement the following steps: 1. **Immediate Communication:** The participant raises their hand and communicates their discomfort, using the pre-established safe word if necessary. 2. **Group Pause:** The group halts all activities and gathers to discuss the situation. 3. **Position Change:** Together, they explore alternative positions that relieve the strain on the participant's back, allowing them to continue participating comfortably. 4. **Incorporating Aftercare:** After the encounter, the group engages in aftercare, including gentle stretches and hydration, to ensure the participant feels supported and cared for.

Conclusion

Addressing physical discomfort and potential injuries in group sexual encounters is vital for fostering a safe and enjoyable atmosphere. By prioritizing communication, employing preventative measures, and responding effectively to discomfort, participants can enhance their collective experience, ensuring that pleasure remains the primary focus. Remember, a well-informed and attentive group is key to navigating the waves of group sexual encounters with confidence and joy.

Incorporating Sensual Touch and Cuddling in Aftercare

After a group sexual encounter, the importance of aftercare cannot be overstated. It is a time for participants to reconnect, process the experience, and nurture the emotional and physical bonds formed during the encounter. One of the most effective ways to achieve this is through sensual touch and cuddling, which can significantly enhance feelings of safety, intimacy, and connection.

The Importance of Sensual Touch

Sensual touch is not merely physical; it is a powerful form of communication that conveys affection, reassurance, and support. Research shows that physical touch can release oxytocin, often referred to as the "love hormone," which promotes bonding and reduces stress. In the context of aftercare, incorporating sensual touch serves several purposes:

+ **Reinforces Connection:** Gentle, affectionate touch helps to reinforce the emotional connections established during the encounter. It fosters a sense of belonging and intimacy, which can be particularly important in group scenarios where participants may have varying degrees of emotional investment.

+ **Facilitates Emotional Processing:** After an intense experience, individuals may need time to process their emotions. Touch can act as a grounding mechanism, helping participants feel more present and connected to their bodies, thereby facilitating emotional processing.

+ **Promotes Relaxation:** Cuddling and gentle caresses can help alleviate any post-play anxiety or discomfort. The soothing nature of touch encourages relaxation and can help participants transition from a heightened state of arousal to a calm and centered state.

Techniques for Sensual Touch

Incorporating sensual touch into aftercare can be approached in various ways. Here are some techniques that can enhance the aftercare experience:

1. **Cuddling:** Simply lying together in a comfortable position can be incredibly nurturing. Participants may choose to spoon, lie face-to-face, or even create a cozy pile of bodies. The key is to find a position that feels safe and comfortable for everyone involved.

2. **Gentle Massage:** Offering a light, sensual massage can help participants release any lingering tension. Focus on areas that may hold stress, such as the shoulders, neck, and back. Use slow, deliberate movements to create a calming effect.

3. **Skin-to-Skin Contact:** Encourage skin-to-skin contact, as it can amplify feelings of intimacy. This can be achieved through simple gestures like holding hands, intertwining fingers, or resting a hand on a partner's back or thigh.

4. **Breath Synchronization:** Engage in breath synchronization exercises, where participants focus on breathing together. This practice can deepen the sense of connection and help regulate emotions. A simple technique is to inhale for a count of four, hold for four, and exhale for six, encouraging a shared rhythm.

5. **Affirmations and Words of Comfort:** While engaging in touch, verbal reassurances can enhance the experience. Participants can express gratitude, share what they enjoyed about the encounter, or simply affirm each other's feelings. This verbal connection can deepen the emotional bond.

Addressing Potential Issues

While incorporating sensual touch and cuddling can be beneficial, it is essential to be mindful of potential issues that may arise:

+ **Differing Comfort Levels:** Not all participants may feel comfortable with touch immediately after a group encounter. It is crucial to check in with each other and establish consent for aftercare practices. Encourage open communication about what feels good and what might be overwhelming.

+ **Processing Emotions:** Some individuals may experience a range of emotions post-play, including vulnerability, sadness, or even regret. It is vital to create a safe space for these feelings to be expressed. Encourage participants to share their emotions openly, and be prepared to listen without judgment.

+ **Physical Discomfort:** After intense physical activity, some participants may feel sore or uncomfortable. Be attentive to each other's physical states and adjust touch accordingly. Gentle, non-intrusive touch can help alleviate discomfort without exacerbating it.

Example Scenario

Consider a scenario where a group of four individuals has just engaged in a fulfilling sexual encounter. As they lie together in a comfortable space, one participant suggests they take a moment for aftercare. They begin by forming a circle, lying on their sides, facing each other.

One person initiates gentle back rubs, while another softly strokes a partner's arm. They take turns sharing what they enjoyed about the encounter, reinforcing positive feelings and affirming each other's experiences. As they engage in this intimate exchange, they synchronize their breathing, creating a shared rhythm that fosters connection.

This example illustrates how simple acts of touch and communication can significantly enhance the aftercare experience, allowing participants to feel safe, cherished, and connected.

Conclusion

Incorporating sensual touch and cuddling into aftercare is a vital practice that enhances emotional intimacy and connection among participants in group sexual encounters. By fostering a nurturing environment through touch, individuals can process their experiences, reinforce bonds, and cultivate a sense of safety and belonging. Emphasizing open communication and consent is essential to ensure that every participant feels comfortable and valued during this intimate time. Ultimately, prioritizing aftercare can transform the overall experience, leading to deeper connections and greater satisfaction in future encounters.

Navigating Potential Fatigue and Energy Drain after Group Play

Group sexual encounters can be exhilarating and deeply fulfilling, but they can also leave participants feeling fatigued or drained. Understanding the physiological and emotional dynamics at play can help you navigate this post-play fatigue effectively. This section explores the causes of fatigue, strategies for recovery, and the importance of self-care in maintaining your sexual health and well-being.

Understanding Fatigue in Group Scenarios

Fatigue after group sexual encounters can stem from various factors, including physical exertion, emotional intensity, and sensory overload. Engaging in multiple sexual activities, particularly in a stimulating environment, can lead to a significant drain on your energy reserves.

Physiological Factors During sexual activity, the body undergoes various physiological changes. Heart rate increases, blood flow intensifies, and hormones like adrenaline and oxytocin surge. These changes are part of the body's natural response to arousal and orgasm, but they also contribute to physical fatigue. Prolonged or intense sexual activity can lead to muscle fatigue, dehydration, and even soreness.

Emotional and Psychological Factors The emotional intensity of group encounters can also contribute to feelings of fatigue. Engaging with multiple partners and navigating complex dynamics can be both exhilarating and exhausting. The release of oxytocin during intimate moments fosters emotional bonding, which can leave you feeling vulnerable or emotionally drained after the experience.

Recognizing Signs of Fatigue

Being attuned to your body and emotions is crucial in recognizing signs of fatigue. Some common indicators include:

+ Physical exhaustion: Muscle soreness, fatigue, and lethargy.

+ Emotional depletion: Feelings of vulnerability, sadness, or irritability.

+ Cognitive overload: Difficulty concentrating or processing thoughts.

+ Sensory overwhelm: Heightened sensitivity to touch, sound, or light.

Recognizing these signs is the first step toward effective recovery.

Strategies for Recovery

Once you identify feelings of fatigue, it's essential to implement strategies for recovery. Here are several effective approaches:

1. Hydration and Nutrition   Replenishing fluids is vital after group play. Sexual activity can lead to significant fluid loss, especially through sweat. Aim to hydrate with water or electrolyte-rich drinks. Additionally, consuming a balanced meal or snack rich in proteins, healthy fats, and carbohydrates can help restore energy levels. For example, a smoothie with banana, spinach, and protein powder can provide quick energy and nutrients.

2. Rest and Relaxation   Allowing your body to rest is crucial. Engage in restorative activities such as gentle stretching, yoga, or simply lying down in a comfortable position. Consider incorporating mindfulness or meditation practices to help calm your mind and body. Techniques such as deep breathing can facilitate relaxation and promote recovery.

3. Sensual Aftercare   Engaging in sensual aftercare can help reconnect with your body and partners. This may include cuddling, gentle touch, or sharing intimate conversations. Such practices not only foster emotional connection but also promote the release of oxytocin, aiding in emotional recovery.

4. Self-Reflection   Post-play reflection can be beneficial. Take time to journal your experiences, noting what felt pleasurable and what may have been overwhelming. This practice can help you process emotions and prepare for future encounters.

The Importance of Self-Care

Self-care is a vital component of navigating fatigue after group play. Prioritizing your well-being not only enhances your recovery but also supports your ongoing sexual exploration. Here are some self-care practices to consider:

- **Mindfulness Practices:** Engage in mindfulness techniques to stay present and grounded. This can include meditation, deep breathing exercises, or guided imagery.

- **Physical Care:** Take a warm bath or shower to soothe sore muscles. Incorporating Epsom salts can further aid relaxation and recovery.

- **Emotional Check-Ins:** Schedule time to check in with yourself emotionally. Consider reaching out to partners for post-play conversations to discuss feelings and experiences.

- **Creative Outlets:** Engaging in creative activities such as art, writing, or music can provide an emotional release and foster healing.

Conclusion

Navigating potential fatigue and energy drain after group sexual encounters is an essential aspect of maintaining your sexual health and well-being.   By understanding the physiological and emotional factors at play, recognizing signs of fatigue, and implementing effective recovery strategies, you can ensure that your experiences remain pleasurable and fulfilling. Embrace self-care as a vital part of your journey, allowing it to enhance your connection with yourself and your partners in future encounters.

Remember, pleasure is not solely found in the act itself, but in the holistic experience that encompasses emotional, physical, and mental well-being.   By honoring your body and emotions, you pave the way for deeper connections and more fulfilling sexual experiences in group settings.

Practicing Hydration and Replenishment of Body Fluids

In the context of group sexual encounters, maintaining proper hydration and replenishing body fluids is essential for both physical comfort and optimal sexual performance. Engaging in intense physical activity, such as sexual play, can lead to significant fluid loss through sweat, increased respiration, and even bodily fluids exchanged during sexual activities. This section will explore the importance of hydration, the physiological impacts of dehydration, and practical strategies for ensuring adequate fluid intake before, during, and after group encounters.

The Importance of Hydration

Hydration plays a crucial role in maintaining bodily functions, including temperature regulation, joint lubrication, and nutrient transport. During sexual activities, the body can lose fluids rapidly, which may lead to dehydration if not adequately addressed. Dehydration can manifest in various ways, including:

+ **Physical Symptoms:** Fatigue, dizziness, dry mouth, and headaches.

+ **Sexual Performance:** Decreased libido, erectile dysfunction, and reduced vaginal lubrication.

+ **Emotional Well-being:** Increased irritability, anxiety, and reduced overall mood.

Physiological Impact of Dehydration

The human body is composed of approximately 60% water, and maintaining this balance is vital for optimal physiological function. Dehydration can lead to an increase in blood viscosity, which can strain the cardiovascular system, making it harder for the body to circulate blood effectively. This is particularly important during sexual arousal, as blood flow to the genitals increases significantly.

The following equation illustrates the relationship between hydration levels and blood volume:

$$\text{Blood Volume} = \text{Total Body Water} \times \text{Blood Volume Fraction} \quad (29)$$

Where the blood volume fraction is typically around 7% of total body weight. A decrease in total body water due to dehydration can significantly reduce blood volume, impacting sexual function and pleasure.

Recommended Fluid Intake

To counteract fluid loss during group sexual encounters, it is essential to have a hydration strategy in place. The general recommendation for daily fluid intake is approximately 3.7 liters for men and 2.7 liters for women, which includes all beverages and food moisture. However, during sexual activities, it is advisable to increase this intake based on individual needs and activity levels.

- **Pre-Encounter Hydration:** Aim to consume an additional 500 mL to 1 liter of water in the hours leading up to the encounter.

- **During the Encounter:** Keep water or electrolyte-rich drinks accessible for sips between activities.

- **Post-Encounter Replenishment:** After the encounter, aim for at least 1 liter of fluid to replenish lost fluids.

Types of Fluids for Replenishment

Not all fluids are created equal when it comes to rehydration. Here are some effective options:

- **Water:** The best option for hydration without added sugars or calories.

- **Electrolyte Drinks:** Beverages containing sodium, potassium, and magnesium can help replenish lost electrolytes, especially after intense activity.

- **Coconut Water:** A natural source of electrolytes that can be refreshing and hydrating.

- **Herbal Teas:** Non-caffeinated herbal teas can provide hydration and have calming effects.

Practical Strategies for Hydration During Group Encounters

To ensure that hydration is prioritized during group sexual encounters, consider the following strategies:

- **Create a Hydration Station:** Set up a designated area with water and electrolyte drinks easily accessible to all participants.

- **Incorporate Breaks:** Plan for short breaks during play to hydrate and check in with each other.

- **Use Visual Reminders:** Place water bottles in visible locations to encourage frequent sipping.

- **Encourage Communication:** Foster an environment where participants feel comfortable reminding each other to hydrate.

Conclusion

Practicing hydration and replenishment of body fluids is a vital aspect of enhancing pleasure and performance during group sexual encounters. By understanding the importance of fluid intake, recognizing the physiological impacts of dehydration, and implementing practical strategies for hydration, participants can ensure a more enjoyable and fulfilling experience. Remember, staying hydrated is not just about physical health; it's also about nurturing emotional well-being and maximizing pleasure in every intimate encounter. So, raise your glass and toast to hydration—your body will thank you!

Engaging in Self-Care Activities for Emotional Well-being

After an exhilarating group sexual encounter, it is essential to prioritize self-care activities that nurture both emotional and physical well-being. Engaging in self-care not only aids in recovery but also enhances emotional resilience, allowing individuals to process their experiences in a healthy manner. This section explores various self-care practices that can be beneficial after group play.

The Importance of Self-Care

Self-care is a multifaceted concept that encompasses a range of activities aimed at promoting health and well-being. According to the World Health Organization (WHO), self-care is defined as the ability of individuals, families, and communities to promote health, prevent disease, and maintain health during illness. After engaging in group sexual encounters, individuals may experience a myriad of emotions, from elation to vulnerability, necessitating a structured approach to self-care.

Common Emotional Responses Post-Encounter

Following group encounters, participants might encounter several emotional responses, including:

- **Euphoria:** A heightened sense of pleasure and connection.

- **Vulnerability:** Feelings of exposure or insecurity.

- **Jealousy:** Comparisons with others or feelings of inadequacy.

- **Sadness:** A sense of loss or emotional letdown after the intensity of the experience.

- **Confusion:** Mixed feelings about the encounter and its implications for personal relationships.

Recognizing these emotions is the first step in engaging in effective self-care.

Self-Care Activities

Here are several self-care activities that individuals can engage in post-group encounter:

1. Reflection and Journaling Taking time to reflect on the experience can be incredibly beneficial. Journaling allows individuals to articulate their thoughts and feelings, providing clarity and understanding. Writing prompts may include:

- What did I enjoy most about the encounter?

- What emotions did I experience during and after the play?

- How did my boundaries hold up, and what could I improve for next time?

This practice not only aids in emotional processing but also fosters personal growth.

2. Mindfulness and Meditation   Mindfulness practices, such as meditation or deep-breathing exercises, can help ground individuals after an intense experience. Engaging in mindfulness allows one to reconnect with their body and emotions, promoting relaxation and reducing anxiety. A simple mindfulness exercise might include:

1. Find a quiet space and sit comfortably.

2. Close your eyes and focus on your breath.

3. Inhale deeply through your nose for a count of four, hold for a count of four, and exhale through your mouth for a count of six.

4. Repeat this cycle for five to ten minutes, allowing thoughts to come and go without judgment.

3. Physical Self-Care   Physical self-care is equally important.   Engaging in activities that promote physical well-being can enhance mood and foster a sense of accomplishment. Consider:

+ **Gentle Exercise:** Activities such as yoga or stretching can alleviate tension and promote relaxation.

+ **Warm Baths:** A warm bath with Epsom salts can soothe sore muscles and provide a calming environment.

+ **Healthy Eating:** Nourishing the body with wholesome foods can improve mood and energy levels.

4. Connecting with Supportive Friends   Reaching out to trusted friends or partners can provide emotional support and validation. Sharing experiences and feelings can alleviate feelings of isolation. Consider arranging a casual get-together or engaging in a comforting activity, such as watching a movie or cooking together.

5. Engaging in Creative Outlets   Creative expression can be a powerful tool for processing emotions.   Activities such as painting, dancing, or crafting can help channel feelings into something tangible. Engaging in creativity allows individuals to explore and express their emotions in a non-verbal manner.

Integrating Self-Care into Routine

To ensure that self-care becomes a regular part of one's life, it is essential to integrate these practices into daily routines. Consider creating a self-care schedule that includes:

+ Daily reflection or journaling sessions.

+ Regular mindfulness or meditation practices.

+ Weekly physical activities that promote well-being.

+ Scheduled time for social connections and creative pursuits.

Conclusion

Engaging in self-care activities after group sexual encounters is crucial for emotional well-being and recovery. By recognizing and addressing emotional responses through reflection, mindfulness, physical care, social connection, and creative expression, individuals can foster resilience and enhance their overall sexual health. Prioritizing self-care not only enriches personal experiences but also contributes to healthier, more fulfilling relationships with oneself and others.

Body Positivity and Self-Appreciation Exercises after Group Scenarios

In the wake of exhilarating group sexual encounters, it's essential to embrace body positivity and self-appreciation. These practices not only enhance your emotional well-being but also foster a healthier relationship with your body, especially after exposing it to the vulnerability of shared intimacy. Here, we will explore various exercises and techniques to cultivate a positive self-image and celebrate your body.

Understanding Body Positivity

Body positivity is the acceptance of all bodies, regardless of size, shape, or appearance. It encourages individuals to appreciate their bodies for what they can do rather than how they look. This movement is crucial in countering societal pressures and unrealistic beauty standards that often leave individuals feeling inadequate or ashamed.

Theoretical Framework The body positivity movement is rooted in several psychological theories, including:

- **Social Comparison Theory:** This theory posits that individuals determine their own social and personal worth based on how they stack up against others. In group sexual encounters, this can lead to feelings of inadequacy if one compares themselves unfavorably to others.

- **Cognitive Dissonance:** When individuals engage in behaviors (like group sex) that contradict their self-image, it can create discomfort. Engaging in self-appreciation exercises can help resolve this dissonance.

- **Self-Compassion:** This concept, developed by Kristin Neff, emphasizes treating oneself with kindness and understanding rather than harsh judgment. Practicing self-compassion is vital for fostering body positivity.

Common Problems Encountered

After group sexual encounters, individuals may experience:

- **Negative Self-Talk:** Criticism of one's body or performance can overshadow positive experiences.

- **Comparison:** Comparing oneself to others in the group can lead to feelings of inadequacy or jealousy.

- **Emotional Vulnerability:** The intimacy of group play can leave individuals feeling exposed, leading to self-doubt.

Self-Appreciation Exercises

To combat these issues, here are some practical exercises to enhance body positivity and self-appreciation:

1. Mirror Work

- Stand in front of a mirror, naked or in comfortable clothing.

- Take a moment to observe your body without judgment.

- Begin to speak positively about your body. For example, "I love my legs for their strength" or "I appreciate my curves and how they feel."

+ Aim to express at least five affirmations. This practice can help rewire negative thought patterns and foster appreciation.

2. Gratitude Journaling

+ Dedicate a journal to body appreciation.

+ Each day, write down three things you are grateful for about your body. For instance, "I am grateful for my hands that create and touch" or "I appreciate my body for its ability to experience pleasure."

+ Reflecting on these aspects can shift focus from perceived flaws to strengths.

3. Movement and Dance

+ Engage in a movement practice that feels good, such as dancing, yoga, or any form of exercise that allows you to connect with your body.

+ Focus on how your body feels during movement rather than how it looks. Celebrate your body's capabilities, its rhythm, and its energy.

+ Consider putting on music that makes you feel empowered and dance freely, embracing every curve and contour.

4. Affirmative Mantras

+ Create a list of affirmations that resonate with you. Examples include:

    – "My body is a vessel of pleasure and joy."

    – "I honor my body and its unique beauty."

    – "I am worthy of love and pleasure, just as I am."

+ Repeat these mantras daily, especially after group encounters, to reinforce a positive self-image.

5. Community Sharing

+ Engage with friends or partners who share similar values about body positivity.

+ Create a safe space to discuss your experiences, feelings, and thoughts about body image.

+ Sharing stories can foster connection and remind you that you are not alone in your feelings.

Integrating Practices into Daily Life

Incorporating these practices into your daily routine is crucial for lasting change. Consider setting reminders on your phone for gratitude journaling or mirror work. Make it a habit to practice self-appreciation regularly, not just after group encounters, to build resilience against negative thoughts.

Conclusion

Embracing body positivity and self-appreciation after group sexual encounters is vital for emotional health and well-being. By engaging in these exercises, individuals can cultivate a loving relationship with their bodies, transforming vulnerability into empowerment. Remember, your body is a magnificent instrument of pleasure and connection, deserving of love and appreciation in all its forms.

Maintaining Connection and Checking in with Group Partners after Play

After an exhilarating group sexual encounter, it's essential to prioritize the emotional and relational dynamics that follow. Maintaining connection and checking in with group partners is not just a courtesy; it's a critical component of fostering trust, intimacy, and emotional safety in group scenarios. This section delves into the significance of post-play check-ins, explores common challenges, and provides practical strategies for nurturing connections after the intensity of shared pleasure.

The Importance of Post-Play Check-Ins

Engaging in group sexual encounters can evoke a wide range of emotions, from euphoria to vulnerability. The aftermath of such experiences often requires reflection and communication to ensure that all participants feel valued and understood. According to attachment theory, the bonds we form with others can significantly influence our emotional well-being. Secure attachment fosters a sense of safety and trust, which is crucial in the context of group play.

$$\text{Emotional Safety} = \text{Trust} + \text{Open Communication} \qquad (30)$$

This equation underscores the idea that emotional safety is a product of trust and open communication. When partners feel safe, they are more likely to express their feelings, concerns, and desires openly, leading to a more satisfying and connected group dynamic.

Common Challenges in Post-Play Communication

Despite the benefits of checking in, participants may face several challenges:

- **Vulnerability:** After an intimate encounter, individuals may feel exposed or insecure about their performance or the dynamics of the group.

- **Jealousy and Insecurity:** Participants may grapple with feelings of jealousy or inadequacy, especially if they perceive a stronger connection between other partners.

- **Fear of Conflict:** Some may avoid post-play discussions out of fear that it could lead to conflict or uncomfortable revelations.

- **Miscommunication:** Without clear communication, misunderstandings can arise, leading to hurt feelings or resentment.

Recognizing these challenges is the first step towards addressing them effectively.

Strategies for Effective Check-Ins

To foster connection and ensure that all partners feel heard and respected, consider the following strategies:

1. **Establish a Check-In Protocol:** Before engaging in group play, discuss how and when to check in afterward. This could be a brief conversation immediately after or a more in-depth discussion within a few days. Setting expectations helps normalize the process.

2. **Create a Safe Space for Sharing:** Encourage an environment where all participants feel comfortable expressing their thoughts and feelings. This can be achieved by using "I" statements, such as "I felt really connected during the experience," which fosters a non-confrontational atmosphere.

3. **Practice Active Listening:** When partners share their feelings, practice active listening by giving them your full attention. Reflect back what you hear to ensure understanding. For example, "It sounds like you felt a bit overwhelmed during the encounter. Can you tell me more about that?"

4. **Address Feelings of Jealousy:** If jealousy arises, approach the topic with sensitivity. Acknowledge the feelings without judgment and explore the underlying causes. For instance, "I noticed you seemed a bit distant during the play. Is there something on your mind?"

5. **Provide Affirmation and Support:** Reinforce the emotional bonds by expressing appreciation for each partner's contributions to the experience. Simple affirmations like, "I really enjoyed the way you engaged with everyone," can help strengthen connections.

6. **Schedule Follow-Up Conversations:** Consider scheduling follow-up conversations to revisit feelings and experiences. This ongoing dialogue can help partners process their emotions over time and reinforce the sense of community within the group.

Examples of Post-Play Check-Ins

To illustrate how these strategies can be applied in practice, consider the following scenarios:

+ **Scenario 1:** After a group encounter, partners gather for a casual debrief. One partner shares, "I felt a little left out at times." The group responds by discussing ways to ensure everyone feels included in future encounters, fostering a sense of teamwork and collaboration.

+ **Scenario 2:** A participant expresses feelings of jealousy regarding another partner's connection with someone else. The group discusses these feelings openly, allowing the jealous partner to express their concerns while others reassure them of their value within the group.

+ **Scenario 3:** Following a particularly intense session, partners agree to check in via a group chat. They share their highlights and any discomforts experienced, promoting ongoing dialogue and support.

Conclusion

Maintaining connection and checking in with group partners after play is an essential practice that contributes to the overall health of the group dynamic. By prioritizing open communication, addressing challenges, and implementing effective strategies, partners can deepen their emotional bonds and enhance their collective experiences. Remember, the goal is not just to enjoy the physical pleasures of group encounters, but to cultivate a rich tapestry of emotional intimacy that supports all participants in their sexual journeys.

$$\text{Connection} = \text{Communication} + \text{Empathy} + \text{Trust} \tag{31}$$

This equation emphasizes that connection is built on the foundations of communication, empathy, and trust, which are vital for nurturing relationships in any sexual context, especially in group scenarios.

Integrating the Experience into Personal Sexual Growth and Exploration

Group sexual encounters can be transformative experiences, offering profound opportunities for personal sexual growth and exploration. After participating in such events, it is essential to take time to reflect on the experience, allowing for deeper integration of the feelings, sensations, and insights gained. This section provides a framework for understanding how to effectively integrate these experiences into your personal sexual journey.

The Importance of Reflection

Reflection is a critical component of personal growth. It allows individuals to process their experiences, understand their reactions, and identify areas for future exploration. To facilitate this process, consider the following reflective practices:

- **Journaling:** Write about your experiences in detail, focusing on your feelings, thoughts, and any new desires that emerged. This practice can help clarify your understanding and solidify your insights.

- **Discussion:** Engage in open conversations with trusted partners or friends about your experience. This dialogue can provide new perspectives and enhance emotional connections.

- **Meditation:** Use mindfulness or meditation techniques to center yourself and process your experiences. This can help in recognizing any lingering emotions and integrating them into your self-awareness.

Identifying Growth Areas

After reflection, identify specific areas for personal growth. This could include:

+ **Desire Exploration:** Did you discover new desires or fantasies during your group encounter? Consider how you can explore these further, whether through solo exploration or with partners.

+ **Communication Skills:** Evaluate how effectively you communicated your needs and boundaries. Identify any challenges you faced and consider strategies for improving your communication in future encounters.

+ **Emotional Awareness:** Reflect on your emotional responses during the encounter. Were there moments of jealousy, insecurity, or unexpected joy? Understanding these feelings can help you navigate them in future situations.

Setting Future Intentions

With insights gained from reflection and identification of growth areas, set clear intentions for your future sexual experiences. Intentions can guide your exploration and help you stay aligned with your evolving desires. Consider the following:

+ **Exploration Goals:** Define what you want to explore next. This could be trying new activities, deepening connections with certain partners, or experimenting with different group dynamics.

+ **Boundaries and Limits:** Reassess your boundaries based on your recent experiences. Are there new limits you wish to establish, or are there areas where you feel ready to expand your comfort zone?

+ **Emotional Growth:** Commit to working on emotional aspects that surfaced during your encounters, such as jealousy or trust issues. This could involve seeking therapy, reading relevant literature, or participating in workshops.

Creating a Personal Growth Plan

To facilitate ongoing sexual growth, create a structured plan that includes:

+ **Regular Check-Ins:** Schedule periodic reflections to assess your progress and make adjustments to your goals as needed.

+ **Engagement with Communities:** Join workshops, online forums, or local meetups focused on sexual exploration and personal development to share experiences and learn from others.

- **Continued Education:** Invest time in reading books, attending seminars, or taking courses that expand your understanding of sexuality, consent, and emotional intelligence.

Embracing a Growth Mindset

Adopting a growth mindset is essential in the journey of sexual exploration. Embrace the idea that experiences—both positive and challenging—contribute to your growth. Remember that:

$$\text{Growth} = \text{Reflection} + \text{Action} + \text{Learning} \tag{32}$$

This equation underscores that growth is not merely a product of experiences but also of how we reflect on and act upon them.

Conclusion

Integrating your group sexual experiences into your personal sexual growth is a dynamic process that enriches your understanding of yourself and your desires. By engaging in reflection, identifying growth areas, setting intentions, and creating a personal growth plan, you empower yourself to navigate future encounters with confidence and clarity. Embrace the journey, and remember that each experience contributes to your unique sexual narrative, fostering a deeper connection to yourself and your partners.

Index